EMPATH & PSYCHIC ABILITIES

THE ESSENTIAL GUIDE TO DEVELOPING YOUR INTUITION, PROTECTING YOUR ENERGY & THRIVING AS A SENSITIVE PERSON IN AN OVERSTIMULATING WORLD

VICA MAYA

© **Copyright by Vica Maya 2022 - All rights reserved.**

The content contained within this book may not be reproduced, duplicated or transmitted without direct written permission from the author or the publisher.

Under no circumstances will any blame or legal responsibility be held against the publisher, or author, for any damages, reparation, or monetary loss due to the information contained within this book. Either directly or indirectly. You are responsible for your own choices, actions, and results.

<u>Legal Notice:</u>

This book is copyright protected. This book is for personal use only. You cannot amend, distribute, sell, use, quote or paraphrase any part, or the content within this book, without the consent of the author or publisher.

<u>Disclaimer Notice:</u>

Please note the information contained within this document is for educational and entertainment purposes only. All effort has been executed to present accurate, up to date, and reliable, complete information. No warranties of any kind are declared or implied. Readers acknowledge that the author is not engaging in the rendering of legal, financial, medical or professional advice. The content within this book has been derived from various sources. Please consult a licensed professional before attempting any techniques outlined in this book.

By reading this document, the reader agrees that under no circumstances is the author responsible for any losses, direct or indirect, which are incurred as a result of the use of the information contained within this document, including, but not limited to — errors, omissions, or inaccuracies.

To my little superheros,

I'm so proud of the sensitive and empathetic people you are growing up to be. May you always embrace your superpowers and use them to make the world a better place. I know you will do amazing things.

Love, Mama

CONTENTS

Join Our Online Community   vii
Introduction   ix

1. UNDERSTANDING EMPATHS   1
   Each Empath is Unique   2
   Signs You Are an Empath   8
   Are Empaths Born or Made?   14
   Empath vs. Highly Sensitive Person   19

2. LIVING LIFE AS AN EMPATH   21
   Benefits of Being an Empath   21
   Overcoming Challenges   29
   Common Myths About Empaths   31

3. DEMYSTIFYING PSYCHIC ABILITIES   35
   Different Types of Psychic Abilities   37
   Empaths and Psychic Abilities   41
   Misconceptions About Psychic Powers   43
   Your Intuition is a Sacred Gift   44
   Ethics and Responsibilities   48

4. HOW TO HEAL AND PROTECT YOUR ENERGY   51
   Meditation For Cleansing your Energy   53
   Using Breath to Change Your Life   55
   White Light Protection   58
   Grounding Your Energy   60
   Setting Energetic Boundaries   61
   Shielding Your Energy   67
   Nature Heals and Restores   68

5. SELF-CARE FOR EMPATHS — 71
   Let's Get Physical! — 71
   Nourishing Your Body — 72
   Water Is the Elixir of Life — 74
   Improving Sleep Quality — 77
   The Magic Power of Crystals — 79
   Essential Oils to Raise Your Vibration — 91
   Create a Sanctuary That Supports You — 103
   Make a Vision Board that Works — 109

6. BALANCING YOUR CHAKRAS — 112
   Exploring the 7 Chakras — 113
   How Chakras Affect Your Intuition — 126
   Chakra Balancing Techniques — 128

7. CONNECTING WITH YOUR INNER WISDOM — 137
   The Magic of Automatic Writing — 140
   Learning to Read Auras — 142
   Connecting With Your Spirit Guides — 146
   Asking for Signs — 150

   CONCLUSION — 153
   LET'S CONNECT! — 157
   Bibliography — 159

JOIN OUR ONLINE COMMUNITY

Join our Facebook group to connect with empaths from all over the world who are dedicated to learning, developing, and empowering one another.

INTRODUCTION

"You're too sensitive!"

"You're so emotional!"

"Stop caring so much!"

If you're an empath, you've probably heard this your whole life. And it's probably something that you're extremely tired of hearing. We live in a world that is constantly telling us to toughen up, not be so sensitive, and just get over it.

I recall my elementary school teachers encouraging me to stop being so "sensitive" when other kids would bother me. Or, as a teenager, my friends would tell me that I was "too emotional" if I cried over a romance movie. And, as an adult, I've been told more times than I can count to just "ignore it" whenever something doesn't sit right with me.

The message was always clear: Being sensitive is not okay.

But here's the thing: Being an empath isn't something that you can just turn off. There's no switch that you can flip to make it all go away. It's hardwired into your very being, an integral part of who you are. It's not something that you can change about yourself, nor should you. It's simply who you are - and there is nothing wrong with that. It is an amazing gift that needs to be cherished, nurtured, and developed. And it's not that we're weak or too emotional. In fact, quite the opposite is true.

Empaths are some of the strongest people out there, carrying the weight of the world on their shoulders. We're just wired a little differently from most people. And once we understand that, it becomes easier to accept ourselves for who we are and turn our challenges into our biggest strengths.

Believe me when I say it wasn't always easy for me to accept my empathy. For most of my life, I tried to hide my sensitivity. I was ashamed of it and felt like there was something wrong with me. It's not like you grow up with a manual on how to be an empath. I wish I had! I thought that if I could just toughen up and stop being so emotional, then everything would be okay. But that's not how it works. The more I tried to hide my emotions, the more they came out in other ways.

I became a people-pleaser, always putting everyone else's needs before my own. I often felt like a doormat, afraid to speak up for myself or set boundaries in my relationships. And I was a constant worrier, obsessing over every little thing that went wrong in my life. Hiding behind a mask of bravado only made my empathy worse. It led to emotional eating, chronic stress, and a whole host of other habits I used to numb my emotions. I was constantly exhausted, both mentally and physically. My relationships suffered, and I felt disconnected from the world around me as if I didn't belong in "normal society."

If you can relate to this, know that you're not alone. There are millions of us out there, all walking our own unique paths. It wasn't until I started to trust my intuition that I began to heal. It wasn't until I realized that there was nothing wrong with being an empath that I was able to start working with my gifts instead of against them. Once I started embracing my sensitivity, I was able to develop healthy coping mechanisms and set healthy boundaries with others. I also began to attract like-minded spiritual people into my life who supported and validated my experience.

Now if someone tells me that I'm being too sensitive, I simply smile and say, "Thank you." It feels so good to finally be at peace with who I am. Why? Because the world needs more empathy. We need more people who are willing to feel, care, and love. We need more people who are willing to be the light in the darkness.

If you're an empath, know that you are a blessing to this world. Your sensitivity is a gift, not a curse. Although I know some days it might feel like one. It is something to be treasured, not hidden away. Know that your sensitivity is a gift—one that can be used to make this world a better place. It's a blessing from the universe that was given to you for a reason. To help you heal the world. To inspire and guide others. To make a difference.

UNDERSTANDING EMPATHS

What does it mean to be an empath? In brief, an empath is someone who is highly sensitive to the emotions and energy of others. Empaths are often described as being "in tune" with the emotions of others, and they can easily take on the emotional state of those around them. They can pick up on the subtlest of cues, and they are very attuned to the nonverbal communication that goes on between people.

It also means that you feel things deeply and profoundly. You have a strong connection to the world around you and can sense the interconnectedness of all things. Empaths are often "old souls" who have a wise and sage-like quality about them. They often see things from a very spiritual perspective and are interested in the deeper questions of life.

EACH EMPATH IS UNIQUE

Empaths are beautiful people who can be found in every walk of life. The term "empath" exists to help us to understand and validate our experiences, but it should not be used as a label to limit our potential. It's important to remember that we are all individuals first and foremost. There are different kinds of empaths and each person has their own unique story, gifts, and talents. See if you can relate to any of the following descriptions:

Emotional Empath

Emotional empaths are people who are highly sensitive to the emotions of others. They can feel what others are feeling, even if they don't show it on the outside. Emotional empaths are often very compassionate and caring. They deeply understand and feel what other people are going through. Emotional empaths often have a strong intuition and can sense when something is wrong.

This is a beautiful gift that allows you to feel the emotions of other individuals and to offer them compassion and understanding. It also means that you are highly sensitive to the energy around you, and you can easily become overwhelmed by it. If you're an emotional empath, it's important to learn how to set boundaries and protect your energy so you can stay healthy and balanced.

Physical Empath

Physical empaths are highly sensitive to the physical sensations of those around them. They can often feel other people's pain in their own bodies, and they can also sense when someone is ill or in danger. For example, if you are a physical empath and you walk into a room where someone has just been arguing, you might feel the tension in the air as if it were your own.

I experience this in the presence of close family members. I can sense when a relative is going through something difficult, even if they don't say anything. And oftentimes, I will start to feel their pain in my own body. It's as if I am feeling it for them.

The other night, I suddenly started feeling sick to my stomach while rocking my baby to sleep. The sensation went away after a few minutes; however, later that night she started throwing up, and I realized she had come down with a stomach bug. She is too young to tell me what was wrong, but my body had picked up on her physical discomfort. Because of empathy, I was able to feel what she was feeling. As a mother, this gift allows me to keep my children safe and to know when they are hurting, even if they can't tell me.

At the same time, it is important for physical empaths to find ways to ground ourselves so that we don't become overwhelmed by the emotions and sensations of those around us.

Intuitive Empath

Intuitive empaths are highly attuned to the thoughts and intentions of others. They can often sense what someone is thinking or feeling, even if that person is trying to hide it. Intuitive empaths are often able to read people's thoughts and intentions, and they can see through deception and lies.

For example, you might be having a conversation with your partner, and you can sense that he is frustrated, even though he is trying not to show it.

You ask him what's wrong, and he insists that everything is fine. But later, he shares with you that he was actually feeling overwhelmed and frustrated. He was trying to hide it because he didn't want to burden you with his problems. That's again empathy at play. You were able to sense what he was feeling, even though he didn't want to make it obvious.

You might also be able to sense what someone is thinking before they even speak. Intuitive empaths often have a strong "gut feeling" about things, and they are usually right. Often blessed with insight, intuitive empaths can help others see the truth that they might be blinded to.

Plant Empath

Plant empaths have a deep connection to the natural world. Plant empaths often have a strong green thumb, although they don't always need to be gardeners to have this gift.

For example, you might be walking through the forest and sense the energy of the plants around you. You might also be able to feel the pain of a tree that is being cut down due to deforestation. It breaks my heart when I see old-growth forests being destroyed.

I can feel the pain of the trees that are being cut down, and it is difficult for me to watch. Plant empaths often have a deep respect for the natural world, and they might feel called to protect the environment.

Animal Empath

Animal empaths have a deep understanding of animal emotions and can often communicate with them on a level that others cannot. They often feel a strong need to protect and care for animals, and they may have difficulty understanding why other people do not feel the same way. Animal empaths are often drawn to careers or initiatives that involve taking care of animals, such as veterinary medicine or animal rescue.

If you have felt a love for animals since you were a child and you're always talking to animals like they were people... chances are, you're an animal empath. You feel like you understand them on a deep level, and they seem to understand you, too. You might even have felt like you were born into the wrong species!

Earth Empath

If you're an earth empath, you probably already know it. Earth empaths are beautiful, sensitive souls who have a deep connection to the planet. They might feel called to protect the earth and its inhabitants. Earth empaths are often passionate about environmentalism or sustainable living.

If you're an earth empath, you might find yourself drawn to nature and the outdoors. You are triggered by the destruction of natural habitats and might feel a need to protect the planet. It hurts you to see the way humans are treating the earth, and you feel a deep need to make a difference.

As an earth empath, you have a responsibility to care for the planet. You might also be interested in sustainability, green living, or permaculture. You can use your gifts to help heal the planet and its inhabitants by working with the earth's energy.

There are many different types of empaths, each with their own unique gifts and abilities. If you recognize yourself in any of these descriptions, there's a good chance you're an empath.

SIGNS YOU ARE AN EMPATH

As you're going through this book, you might be thinking, "This is me a hundred percent. I am DEFINITELY an empath!" Or if this is a new idea to you, you might need more time to process it. That's okay, too. Here are some signs that you might be an empath, even if you're not sure yet:

Do you have a hard time saying no when people ask for favors?

Empaths are often people-pleasers and have a hard time saying no to others, even when they really need to. They care so much about others that they hate to disappoint them. It took me a while to learn that saying no is not only okay, but sometimes it's necessary. You need to take care of your own needs too, and that means setting and respecting your own boundaries.

Do you tend to be a peacekeeper and avoid conflict?

Empaths often avoid conflict because they don't like to see people upset. They will go out of their way to make sure everyone is happy and comfortable. This can be a great trait, but it's important to know when to stand up for yourself. Not every situation warrants peacekeeping, and sometimes you need to voice your own needs and opinions.

Do you feel other people's emotions as if they were your own?

Empaths are highly sensitive to the emotions of others. They can often sense when someone is upset or going through a tough time, even if that person doesn't say anything. They have this magical superpower to read between the lines and see what's really going on.

I often joke that empaths would make the world's best detectives because they just know things. They wouldn't need a badge or years of training to figure out who the bad guy is; they just know. Even if you're not planning to be the next Sherlock Holmes, this ability to read people can be really helpful in all areas of your life. Your intuition, when coupled with logic, can help you navigate the world in a way that others can't.

Do you pick up on the energy of a room as soon as you walk in?

Empaths are very in tune with the energy around them. They can often feel the vibes of a room as soon as they walk in. This applies to both positive and negative energy. Positive energy can be uplifting and make an empath feel happy, while negative energy can be draining and make them feel tired. If you're an empath, you might want to avoid places that are full of negative energy, like crowded bars or busy city streets where there's too much stimulation.

When I was working at my corporate job, I used to take the train to work. There was just too much energy for me to process, and it would leave me feeling exhausted by the time I got to the office. Busy transport hubs are a mecca for mixed energies, so it might be best to avoid them or travel during offpeak times.

Do you have a hard time being around negative people?

Nobody enjoys being around nay-sayers and Debbie Downers, but for empaths, it can be especially draining. Empaths tend to absorb the emotions of those around them, so being around pessimistic people can really bring them down. Often referred to as emotional vampires, negative people can sap the energy of an empath and leave them feeling exhausted. It's important to limit your exposure to these types of people, or at least learn how to protect your energy around them.

If you find yourself avoiding certain individuals because you just can't deal with their negativity, you might be an empath. For years, I thought this was the norm and that everyone felt the same way I did around negative people. It wasn't until I started learning about empathy that I realized how sensitive I was to the energy of others. Hours later, I would still be feeling the effects of a negative encounter, while others seemed to brush it off like it was nothing. If you ever feel drained, like you need a nap after being around someone, you might very well be an empath.

Do you need alone time to recharge?

Empaths need quiet time to recharge their batteries. They can enjoy being around others, but they also need time alone to relax and rejuvenate to feel balanced again. It doesn't necessarily mean that they are introverts, although many empaths are. It just means that they need time alone to process everything that's going on around them.

It's important to note that there's a spectrum when it comes to being an empath. It's not all black and white, and you don't have to check off every single sign to be an empath. For example, I consider myself an extroverted introvert, which means I get my energy from being around people, but I also need time alone to decompress. In other words, don't feel like you need to change who you are to fit some arbitrary definition. Not all empaths are the same, and that's what makes each individual beautiful and unique.

Do you have a hard time watching the news or reading the paper?

Empaths often have a hard time watching the news or reading newspaper headlines because they can't handle seeing all the negative things going on in the world. The media tends to focus on the bad, and for empaths, it can be a lot to process. Empaths can find the news overwhelming and depressing. It's just too much for them to take in.

Cutting out the news and negative people in your life isn't going to make the world's problems go away, but decreasing your exposure will help you to stay focused on the positive and not get overwhelmed. It's important to have control over what you take in, and for empaths, that means being selective about the news you watch and the people you spend your time with.

Do you attract "broken people" into your life?

If you're an empath, you might find that "broken people" are drawn to you. I've heard from so many empaths that they attract people who are going through a tough time in their lives. "I would be shopping for groceries and people would approach and tell me their whole life story. It happens all the time," one woman shared in our chat. "I can't even count the number of times I've had strangers come up to me and start pouring their heart out. It's like they can sense that I'm a good listener," said another empath.

If you find people venting their problems to you, even if you don't know them well, it could be because energetically they sense your empathy and feel safe sharing their stories with you. You might not be able to fix their problems, but your presence and compassion is comforting and healing to them.

The same is true for relationships. If you're an empath, you might find yourself in relationships with people who are needy, or who take advantage of your good nature. For this exact reason, I had to let go of a number of friendships that were no longer serving me. If you find yourself in a one-sided relationship where you're always the one giving and the other person is always taking, it might be time to step back and take a look at the situation. You deserve the same level of care and attention that you're giving to others.

ARE EMPATHS BORN OR MADE?

People can develop their empathy for different reasons. Some are born with the ability to sense and feel the emotions of others, while others develop the ability later in life. Here are five of the most common reasons people become empaths:

Genetics

Empaths are often born into families with other empaths. If you have empathy, there's a good chance that your parents or grandparents were also empaths. In my case, I can see how empathy has been passed down in genetics through my mother. My mom has a beautiful, nurturing soul and has always been a giver. She's an amazing listener and has always been able to provide comfort and support to those who need it. I'm grateful to have her as a role model in my life. In fact, it's because of her unconditional support that I'm writing this book today. Thanks, Mama!

Temperament

Temperament refers to a person's natural disposition or inborn qualities. People with certain personality traits are more likely to develop empathy than others. For example, people who are naturally compassionate, sensitive, and introspective are more likely to develop their spiritual abilities.

If you recall when you were a child, chances are you were already quite sensitive and intuitive. You might have been the one in your class who always comforted the other kids when they were upset. Or you might have been the one who got teased for being "a cry baby" when you got your feelings hurt. If you can relate to any of this, it's likely that you've always been an empath. Some children are born empaths, while others develop their abilities later in life.

Traumatic Life Experiences

Certain individuals develop empathy after experiencing a traumatic event. For example, people who have been through abuse, neglect, or tragedy can sometimes develop empathy as a way to cope with their pain. When we experience trauma, our hearts open in ways that we never thought possible.

We become more compassionate and understanding of the pain of others because we have experienced it ourselves. There's a reason we often hear the expression that some of the most compassionate people are those who have been through the most pain.

Supportive Upbringing

If you were lucky enough to have a supportive and loving upbringing, there's a higher chance you'll develop empathy. When we feel loved and supported, we develop a sense of safety in the world. We feel confident and secure in who we are. This allows us to open our hearts more fully to others. It also allows us to develop our intuitive talents. Having role models in our lives who are empaths can inspire and encourage us to develop and grow.

It could be a parent, grandparent, teacher, or mentor who helps you to develop your empathy. These are the people who see our potential and encourage us to use our gifts. They might even share their own experiences with us and teach us how to use our abilities in helpful ways.

As a parent, I am constantly thinking of how important it is to provide a supportive and loving environment for my children. I want them safe and loved so that they can grow into their full potential and use empathy and intuition in their everyday lives. I hope this book will spark some conversations about empathy in your own family and help us create a more compassionate world for future generations.

Spiritual Awakening

A spiritual awakening can also trigger empathy. Spiritual awakening refers to a process of personal transformation. It's a time when we let go of our old ways of thinking and being and open up to new possibilities. An individual might feel they are awakening to a new level of consciousness and understanding. They may feel a deep connection to the world around them and feel called to help others.

If you find yourself empathizing with people more than ever before, it could be a sign that you are undergoing a spiritual awakening. You might have a sudden desire to help other people or feel called to a higher purpose. You may also feel more connected to the world around you and have a greater understanding of the interconnectedness of all things. As you become more in tune with your own emotions and the emotions of others, you may find yourself being more compassionate and understanding. If you are experiencing a spiritual awakening, it is essential to take care of yourself and keep learning. Seek out supportive people, resources, and environments that will help you grow and thrive.

Regardless of how you became an empath, you are on a spiritual path of growth and expansion.

EMPATH VS. HIGHLY SENSITIVE PERSON

It's important to understand the difference between an empath and a highly sensitive person (HSP). While both of these types are sensitive to the emotions of others, there are some key differences.

Contrary to popular belief, not all empaths are highly sensitive people, but the two do tend to go hand in hand. Empaths are highly attuned to the emotions and energy of others, to the point where they can often absorb and feel these emotions themselves.

HSPs are often highly sensitive to environmental factors such as loud noise, bright lights, and crowds. They might also have a lower pain threshold and be extra sensitive to medications, food additives, and chemicals. HSPs can also be very sensitive to other people's feelings, but they don't necessarily absorb and experience these emotions as their own the same way empaths do.

It's not uncommon for empaths to also be HSPs. In fact, studies have shown that up to seventy percent of HSPs are also empaths. However, it's important to understand the difference between the two terms so that you can better understand how your mind and body work.

Let me share a personal story. The last time I went to the dentist and needed to get a filling, the anesthetic didn't numb my mouth enough. The dentist had to give me two extra doses, and even then I could still feel the drilling. The sound of the drill was also torture. "Wow, you're so sensitive," he said in disbelief. "I've never seen someone react like this before." I just shrugged and said, "I'm used to it," while making a mental note that I'll need to mail him a copy of this book for Christmas!

For me, being an empath and an HSP goes hand in hand. I know I have a lower pain threshold, I'm highly sensitive to sugar and refined foods, and I definitely absorb the emotions of others. As you can see, the difference between being an empath or a highly sensitive person is not black and white. There is a spectrum of sensitivity, and where you fall on that spectrum depends on your unique life experiences, genetics, and abilities.

LIVING LIFE AS AN EMPATH

BENEFITS OF BEING AN EMPATH

Being an empath comes with a lot of responsibility. To thrive as an empath, it is important to be aware of your own needs and boundaries. It can be easy to get overwhelmed by the challenges of the world, but it is also important to remember that you have the power to make a difference, and you were put on this earth for a reason. As the goal of this book is to empower you to use your abilities in positive ways, let's take a look at some of the benefits of being an empath. (These are just a few of many!)

You Are Highly Intuitive

Empaths possess an innate ability to intuit what others are feeling and thinking, and they often have a deep understanding of the human condition. This makes empaths natural healers, loving partners, and supportive friends. This also means that empaths are often very good at reading people. They can quickly pick up on social cues and read between the lines. This intuition can be a great asset in both personal and professional relationships. It helps them navigate difficult conversations and can be used to build trust and rapport in all interactions.

You Are Caring and Compassionate

Because empaths are so aware of others' emotions, they are often very caring and compassionate individuals. They have a deep desire to help others and make the world a better place. They feel the pain of others as if it were their own, and they are often driven to help those who are suffering. That's a lot of weight to carry, but it also means that empaths are some of the strongest people you will ever meet.

This compassion is one of the most beautiful aspects of being an empath. It allows you to connect with others on a deep level and helps you to create lasting bonds. It also gives you the ability to make a ripple effect of positive change in the world. If you're an empath, you may have already found yourself in the role of unofficial counselor to your friends and family. You might be the one everyone comes to for a shoulder to cry on—or for some tough love when they need it. Some may even say that you're wise beyond your years. Your wisdom goes hand in hand with your intuition and allows you to see things that others might miss.

You Have a Creative Spark

Empaths tend to have rich inner worlds, and they are often highly imaginative. This creativity often manifests itself in the arts, but it can also be seen in the way that empaths view the world. Many talented writers, artists, and musicians are empaths. They view the world through a unique lens that allows them to see the beauty in everyday life.

You might feel the desire to express yourself through writing, painting, music, dance, or another creative outlet. And you should! Your talents do not need to be what you do for a living. Nor do you need to be a master of your craft to enjoy the creative process.

Your creative expression can bring joy to others, balance your own energy, and help you to connect with the world in a deeper way. This creativity can also be an asset in more practical pursuits. Empaths are often problem-solvers. They are able to look at a problem from multiple angles and come up with creative solutions.

You Are Aware of Your Surroundings

Empaths understand what motivates people, and they can see through surface-level appearances. They intuitively feel what makes people tick, what cheers them up, and what stresses them out. This ability to understand and connect with others on a spiritual level is one of the empath's most valuable gifts.

Empaths often have a keen awareness of social injustice and inequality, and they are often driven to make a difference in the world. Their heightened awareness can also make empaths excellent observers. They can often sense danger long before it arrives and keep negative situations from happening.

You Are Open-Minded and Accepting

Empaths are often very open-minded and tolerant of others. Sometimes to a fault. They see the world in all its shades of grey, and they are able to find beauty in unexpected places. This open-mindedness can be a great strength, as it allows empaths to connect with people from all walks of life. Because empaths are so non-judgmental, they are able to see the best in people. Even when others can't. For this reason, empaths are often seen as a pillar of unconditional support in their circle of friends. They treat everyone with acceptance and love.

They know that everyone is on their own journey, and they are usually non-judgmental of the choices that others make. This acceptance is one of the things that makes empaths such wonderful people. It allows them to create connections with others that are based on understanding and respect.

You See Both Sides of Every Issue

Because empaths are so aware of others' needs and underlying intentions, they are often able to see both sides of every issue. They understand that there is rarely one right answer and that people often have different perspectives on the same situation. They can easily put themselves in others' shoes and see how they would feel in the same situation.

This ability to see both sides can be a great asset in many areas of life. It allows empaths to be excellent mediators and peacemakers. As leaders, this quality makes them naturally skilled at seeing the potential in others. As team members, they are often able to find common ground and build bridges between opposing viewpoints.

You Are a Great Listener

It should come as no surprise that empaths are excellent listeners. They are usually patient and carefully consider what is being said without judgment. This quality allows empaths to create a safe space for others to express themselves. This is because they understand that everyone has a story to tell and that each person's perspective is valid.

This ability to listen also allows empaths to really hear what others are saying. They can see beyond the surface and tune into the deeper meaning of someone's message. This makes empaths very good at giving advice and support. This is why other people are drawn to them in times of trouble.

You Are a Natural Healer

At a subatomic level, our bodies are made up largely of space. It's the energy that fills that space—the electrons whirling around the nucleus of each atom—that give us mass and form. We are literally beings of energy vibrating at different frequencies. When we experience disharmony in our lives, it's often because our energy is out of balance.

Empaths are natural healers. They have the ability to sense imbalances in other people's energy, and they can help to bring about balance and harmony. They can often sense when someone is off, even if they don't know what's wrong. And they have a natural inclination to want to fix it.

Empaths have the gift of being able to see the world through the lens of energy. They understand that all beings are connected both on a physical and spiritual level. This understanding allows them to have a deep respect for all life, and it is also what makes them natural healers.

You Seek Meaningful Relationships

Empaths are often drawn to relationships that are based on a deep connection and mutual understanding. They usually don't do well in relationships that are based on superficial things like power or money.

This is because empaths understand that relationships are about so much more than just what we can see on the surface. They are about an exchange of energy and a deep connection of the soul. When empaths are in a relationship, they are usually all in. They give their relationships everything they've got.

Empaths usually want their relationships to be meaningful and lasting. They are often attracted to people who are also looking for a deep connection. They get easily bored or disconnected in relationships that are based on anything less.

You Find Beauty in Simplicity

Empaths are often attracted to things that are simple and natural. They appreciate the beauty in everyday moments, and they find joy in the small things.

Empaths are able to find peace and calm in the midst of chaos. This is because they need time to reconnect with their own energy and the energies of the earth. It is in these moments of solitude that empaths are able to recharge and rejuvenate. When out in nature, they can tune out the noise of the world and connect with the peace that lies within. It allows them to appreciate the small things in life, and it also helps them to stay grounded during difficult times.

Empaths are often seen as the healers of the world. And while this is certainly true, it is only a small part of who they are. Empaths are complex and multi-dimensional beings with many gifts and talents. This list is by no means exhaustive. But it does give you a taste of some of the most common empath traits.

Did any of these resonate with you? If yes, it's time to start exploring your own empathic nature. And I'm going to be here to guide you on your journey to self-discovery!

OVERCOMING CHALLENGES

While being an empath comes with many advantages, it also comes with its own set of challenges. I would be lying if I said that being an empath is always easy. It's not. In fact, it can be downright difficult at times.

The challenges of being an empath often arise when they are not able to properly care for themselves. When they don't take the time to recharge and rejuvenate, they can quickly become overwhelmed. This can lead to energy overwhelm, and it can also make them susceptible to negative influences. It's important for empaths to learn how to protect their energy. This is one of the most common challenges that empaths face. Otherwise, they run the risk of becoming overloaded and burned out.

One way to protect your energy is to create boundaries. This means learning to say no when you need to and setting healthy boundaries with people in your life. It also means taking time for yourself and doing things that energize you and make you happy. As the saying goes, you cannot pour from an empty cup. So make sure to take care of yourself first and foremost.

A wonderful way to protect and heal yourself is to surround yourself with positive energy. This includes spending time in nature, listening to uplifting music, and surrounding yourself with love and light. Later in this book, I'll share specific tips and techniques for protecting your energy and grounding yourself.

For now, just know that these are some of the most important things that you can do as an empath. Consider this book a self-care manual of sorts. It's designed to help you care for yourself so that you can enjoy life to the fullest.

COMMON MYTHS ABOUT EMPATHS

As I embarked on my journey of self-discovery, I quickly realized that there were a lot of myths and misconceptions about empaths. Fair enough. I mean, we empaths are a pretty mysterious bunch. But still, it was frustrating to see so many people spreading false information, so I decided to set the record straight in this book.

Myth: Empaths Are Always Nice

First of all, empaths are not always nice. In fact, empaths can be pretty darned moody and opinionated if they get upset. They are also not always gentle, calm, and shy. Empaths can be bold and outspoken when they need to be. Just because empaths are sensitive, it doesn't mean that they don't have their own opinions and views. They're human, after all. Empaths have their good and bad days, just like everyone else.

Myth: Empaths Are Weak

One of the most common myths about empaths is that they are weak. This couldn't be further from the truth! Empaths are some of the strongest and most resilient people on the planet. We have to be in order to deal with the constant barrage of energy that we are bombarded with on a daily basis. So if you're ever feeling down about yourself, just remember that you are strong and capable. Empaths may be emotional, but we are much tougher than we realize.

Myth: Empaths Can See Through People

While it's true that empaths are very intuitive, we don't always know what other people are thinking or feeling. We can usually get a pretty good sense of it, but we are not necessarily mind readers. In situations where emotions are running high, it can be difficult for even the most self-aware empath to discern what's really going on. Sometimes, it can be challenging to differentiate between intuition and projection, but that's all part of being human.

Myth: Empaths Are Always Positive

Empaths are not always happy. In fact, they can be downright crabby at times! They have a lot of emotions to process (their own and other people's). They feel pain, sadness, anger, and frustration just like everyone else. The difference is that empaths feel emotions more intensely than others. So if you're ever feeling low, just know that it's perfectly normal (and even healthy) for empaths to have negative emotions from time to time.

Myth: One Can Stop Being an Empath

This is another myth that I see a lot. People think that empaths can just "turn off" their abilities or stop feeling external energy. You might've heard your friends or family say, "Why can't you just stop taking things so close to heart?"

But the truth is, once you're an empath, you're always an empath. Your empathy doesn't come with a battery-powered remote control! It's not something that you can turn on or off at will.

Although that would be nice, wouldn't it? Instead, what you can do is learn how to control and manage your energy so that it doesn't overwhelm you. Your "remote control" is your ability to set boundaries, say "no," and take care of yourself. By learning how to do these things, you can protect yourself from negative energies and maintain your own sanity!

Myth: Empaths Are Perfect and Better Than Others

Although my intention for this book is to empower empaths and show them what superheroes they are, I want to be clear that empaths are not perfect. There is no place for ego or self-righteousness in empathy. Empaths are simply people who have a special set of talents and need to learn how to use them in a way that is helpful, not harmful to themselves or others.

The bottom line is that empaths are perfectly imperfect, just like everyone else. We have our own unique set of strengths and weaknesses. We're sensitive, but we're also strong. We have good days and bad days. It's all part of being human. And that's something we can all empathize with!

DEMYSTIFYING PSYCHIC ABILITIES

There are two categories of people in the world: those who believe in psychic abilities and those who don't. I used to be somewhere in between—a skeptical believer. That is until I realized I had some of those abilities myself as an empath.

Psychic abilities are real, and they're more common than you might think. They are extrasensory abilities that allow individuals to perceive information beyond the five senses. These skills are often referred to as "ESP," or extrasensory perception. In other words, they enable people to tap into a sixth sense or what is commonly known as intuition.

When some people hear the word "psychic," they envision scenes from movies with a fortune-teller gazing into a crystal ball, smoke swirling around her head, and a black cat perched on her shoulder. Okay, maybe not everyone does this, but I know I did before I knew anything about psychic powers...

But the truth is, psychic abilities come in many different forms, and not all of them are as dramatic or noticeable as Hollywood would have us believe. In fact, most psychics are much more subtle. For example, have you ever had a feeling that someone was going to call you, and then they did? Or have you ever said something out loud at the same time as someone else? These are both examples of psychic abilities in action!

Similar to empathy, it's best to imagine psychic abilities on a spectrum. We all have some degree of psychic ability, some more than others. No matter where they fall on the spectrum, all psychic abilities share one common trait: They all involve the ability to perceive information that is outside of the normal range of human senses. One of the most important things to remember about psychic abilities is that they are natural talents that we all have. We can all develop and strengthen our psychic skills, but some people are more in tune with their abilities than others.

Just like any other talent or skill, the more you practice using your psychic abilities, the stronger they will become. As an empath, you have a head start on developing your abilities, as you are already in touch with your emotions and intuition.

DIFFERENT TYPES OF PSYCHIC ABILITIES

So now that we know what psychic abilities are, let's take a closer look at some of the most common ones. The four main categories of psychic abilities I'd like to highlight are clairvoyance, clairsentience, clairaudience, and claircognizance. If this is all new to you, don't worry! I'll explain what each of these abilities entails.

Clairvoyance

The word "clairvoyant" comes from the French meaning "clear seeing." Clairvoyants might see, hear, feel, or know things that other people cannot. They might see images, symbols, and colors that provide them with information about a person, place, or situation. They can predict future events or get glimpses of potential outcomes.

Clairvoyance is one of the most well-known psychic abilities, but it's also one of the most misunderstood. Many people believe that clairvoyance is all about seeing the future, but this is only a small part of what clairvoyants can do.

Clairvoyance is actually more about using your intuition and "inner knowing" to gain information about people, places, and things. It's about understanding the energy and vibrations that are all around us and using that information to provide insight and guidance. Their visions can help people make decisions, solve problems, and find closure.

Clairsentience

Clairsentience is probably the most common psychic ability among empaths. Clairsentience is the ability to feel or sense energy. This can manifest in many ways, such as feeling someone's presence when they are not there, sensing when something is going to happen, or getting "gut feelings" about people or potential situations.

Clairsentience is a great ability to have if you are looking for guidance from your intuition or Higher Self. Many people use their clairsentience to make decisions in their everyday lives. For example, you might get an uneasy feeling when you meet someone new. This could be your intuition trying to warn you that this person is not to be trusted.

If you trust your gut instinct and listen to your intuition, you will start to notice that your clairsentience will become more accurate over time. The more you practice using your abilities, the stronger they will get.

Clairaudience

Clairaudience is a form of extrasensory perception that allows you to hear things that are not audible to the human ear. As I heard a fellow empath describe it, "It feels like a gentle whisper in my ear," which is quite different from the harsh or tormenting voices experienced by people with psychological conditions, hormonal imbalances, or serious vitamin deficiencies.

The messages you hear can provide support when you need it most. For example, a clairaudient might hear a loved one's voice from the other side or receive guidance from their spirit guide during meditation. If you suspect that you have clairaudience, it's important to trust your intuition and follow your heart. The more you open yourself up to this ability, the more you will be able to receive spiritual guidance.

Claircognizance

Claircognizance is the ability to know things without knowing how you know them. This is often referred to as "inner knowing" or "intuition." Claircognizance is a very powerful ability and can be very helpful in making decisions or gathering information. If you're claircognizant, you may have a strong feeling about which direction to take in your life or a particular course of action, even though you can't explain why.

Before I met my husband, I felt a strong desire to travel across Canada to Montreal, even though I had no logical reason to do so. I even had vivid dreams about going there. This curiosity and inner knowing led me to buy a one-way ticket from Vancouver to Montreal, where I met him at a salsa class one month later. What are the chances? Ten years, two kids, and three cats later, I am so grateful that I followed my intuition!

Claircognizance can also manifest as sudden "downloads" of information or knowledge. This is often how channelers or psychics receive information from their guides or higher selves. If you are claircognizant, you may find that you are able to make decisions quickly, without second-guessing yourself. If you have a strong feeling about something, trust it, and act on it.

As you can see, psychic abilities are varied and complex. But one thing is for sure: We all have them! And we can all develop them with practice. So if you're interested in honing your intuition, follow the exercises in this book and see where they take you. Who knows, you might just surprise yourself!

EMPATHS AND PSYCHIC ABILITIES

Scientifically, we know that energy cannot be created or destroyed. It must go somewhere. Our bodies are made up of atoms, which are in turn made up of protons, neutrons, and electrons. These particles are in a constant state of motion and have a corresponding frequency or vibration. Thanks to my grade 10 biology teacher, I know that the human body is made up of anywhere from 50 to 75 trillion cells. And each one of our cells has a frequency.

What the typical high school textbook fails to mention is that our thoughts and emotions also have a corresponding frequency or vibration. When we think positive thoughts, we emit a high-frequency vibration. When we think negative thoughts, we emit a low-frequency vibration. Those are the basic building blocks of our physical and spiritual reality.

Empaths are highly sensitive to these frequencies and can sense even the subtlest changes. Similar to the way radio can tune into different frequencies, empaths can tune into the thoughts and emotions of others. These vibrations are not visible to the human eye; however, that doesn't mean they don't exist. Empaths have the ability to dial into these frequencies and receive the information they contain. Pretty amazing, isn't it? The ability to sense the energy that is not visible to the eye is nothing short of a superpower.

How amazing will it be when textbooks start teaching this stuff in school? Imagine if we all knew about the Law of Attraction and how to manifest our desires. The world would be a very different place!

MISCONCEPTIONS ABOUT PSYCHIC POWERS

Many people think that psychic abilities are just wishful thinking or hocus pocus. I can't blame them. With the proliferation of fake psychics and mediums, it's no wonder that people are sceptical or even frightened by extrasensory abilities. Media, movies, and television shows have also done a lot to sensationalize psychic abilities, making them seem like something out of a sci-fi movie.

The truth is that psychic abilities are very real, and they are nothing to be afraid of. Many people have these abilities but don't even realize it. If you've ever had a strong gut feeling or knew something was going to happen before it did, then you have experienced a form of psychic ability.

The problem is that many people grow up being told that psychic abilities are fake or evil, so they suppress these abilities and don't allow themselves to develop them. This is nothing new to our society. Centuries ago, back in the days of the Salem witch trials, people with psychic abilities were persecuted and even killed. Thankfully, times have changed, and we are now starting to accept these abilities as natural gifts.

There's a lot of fear and taboo surrounding psychic abilities, yet these powers remain a natural part of who we are. Everyone has intuition; it's just a matter of whether or not we listen to it. If your intuitive abilities are dormant, there are ways to develop them.

The key is not to let the myths and misconceptions about psychic abilities prevent you from exploring your full potential. If you picked up this book, I am willing to bet that you had a hunch that there's more to your potential than what you've been led to believe. I encourage you to explore your talents and see where they take you. Embrace your inner wisdom, and let your intuition guide you on your spiritual journey!

YOUR INTUITION IS A SACRED GIFT

Let's flip the script for a minute. Instead of thinking about psychic abilities as something weird or strange, let's think about them as a sacred gift.

Psychic abilities are simply a heightened form of intuition. Intuition is something that we all have and use on a daily basis. It's that little voice inside our head that tells us when something feels off or warns us of danger. It's also the voice that gives us creative ideas and solutions to problems.

When you tune in to your intuitive abilities, you are tapping into a powerful source of guidance and wisdom, kindness, and compassion. It knows what you need before you do, and it will not steer you wrong. Psychic abilities are simply an extension of this natural intuition that we all possess. When you develop your psychic abilities, you are opening yourself up to even more guidance, creativity, and possibilities.

Intuition is also highly linked to creativity. When you trust your intuition, you are tapping into a well of creativity that is always available to you. Creativity does not mean that you have to wait for inspiration to strike. It is always there, waiting to be accessed. Creativity empowers you to see the world in new ways, become a resourceful problem-solver, and come up with innovative ideas. There is no limit to what you can achieve when you listen to your intuition and trust your inner knowing.

I love the quote by Albert Einstein that goes, "The intuitive mind is a sacred gift, and the rational mind is a faithful servant. We have created a society that honors the servant and has forgotten the gift." Considering Einstein's famously brilliant mind, I think it's safe to say that we should all start listening to our intuition a bit more.

Using Your Powers to Impact the World

Psychic abilities can be used for good or ill, but I believe that we all have the potential to use our abilities to make a positive impact on the world. When we use our psychic abilities for good, we are tapping into a powerful force that can improve lives.

If you are interested in using your abilities to help others, there are many ways to do so. You can use your intuition to help people heal from traumas, give them guidance on their life path, or receive invaluable guidance. When people are at a crossroads in their lives, your intuition can be a powerful tool to help them make decisions. When going through difficulties, people need someone who can offer them hope and compassion. You can use your intuitive abilities to be that person for someone else. You have the power to make a real difference in the world. All it takes is a little bit of courage to step out and use your gifts.

You can also use your intuitive abilities to help animals and the environment. Some of the most caring people I know are intuitive empaths who care for animals in need. They can sense what animals are feeling, which helps them understand what the animals need and how to help them. Many empaths become the voice for animals.

We can also use our psychic abilities to connect with the Earth and sense where there is pollution or environmental damage. We can use them to send healing energy to the Earth and help promote global healing.

Your intuition can also be a powerful gift when it comes to working with children. By tuning into the emotional frequency of a child, empaths can provide guidance and support. They can help a child understand and process their feelings and offer a comforting presence during times of frustration. In addition, psychic empaths can also offer insights into the future. By helping children tap into their own intuition, they can empower them to make choices that are in alignment with their highest good. As more and more children learn to understand and use their empathy and intuition, the world will become a more compassionate and loving place.

When we use our empathy and psychic abilities to help others, we are fulfilling our life purpose. When we use our gifts to make a difference, we are living our truth. So if you're feeling called to make an impact in the world, know that you have everything you need within you to do so. Trust your intuition and follow your heart. The world needs your light.

ETHICS AND RESPONSIBILITIES

This book wouldn't be a complete guide on empathy and psychic abilities if we didn't touch on the ethical and responsible use of these gifts. Just because I have $500 to spend on chocolate cheesecake doesn't mean that I will or should. (Although I must admit, it's tempting!) The same goes for psychic abilities. Just because you can do something doesn't mean that you should do it.

There are certain ethical considerations that need to be taken into account when using your powers. This concept applies to all areas of life, but it's especially important when we're talking about abilities that can impact the lives of others.

When using your psychic abilities, always consider the highest good of all involved. This includes you, the person you are intending to help, and any other beings who may be affected by your actions. It's also important to get consent before using your abilities on someone else. This is a basic principle of respect and consideration. Just as you wouldn't want someone to use their abilities on you without your consent, don't do it to others. If someone doesn't want your insights, honor their wishes and respect their boundaries.

Another important thing to consider is the intention behind your actions. When you use your abilities for the highest good of all involved, you are more likely to experience positive results. However, if you use your abilities with the intention of manipulating or controlling someone, you not only violate their free will, but you are also likely to experience negative consequences. This is because our actions always come back to us, whether we realize it or not. So if you want to use your abilities in a way that is positive and helpful, make sure your intentions are pure.

Remember, your psychic abilities are a gift. They are meant to be used as a tool for healing, growth, and transformation. When used responsibly, they can be a force for good in the world. Always remember to act with integrity, compassion, and respect. These are the cornerstone values of any empath.

As our planet transitions into a more spiritually awake state, the need for ethical and responsible intuitives will become even greater. We are moving into a time when more and more people are going to be looking for spiritual guidance and support. As an empath or psychic, you have the ability to offer them just that.

When we make choices that are in alignment with the highest good, we create a positive ripple effect that can impact the lives of many. A flap of a butterfly's wings can create a hurricane. In the same way, our actions, no matter how small, can have a big impact on the planet.

HOW TO HEAL AND PROTECT YOUR ENERGY

As we go through life, we all accumulate a lot of emotional baggage. Metaphorically speaking, if the aura is a suitcase, then most of us are walking around with one that's overflowing. We're carrying around emotional wounds from our past, trauma from this lifetime and other lifetimes, and energetic debris from the people and places we've known. All of this can weigh us down and make it difficult to live our best lives.

This baggage can affect our energy levels, moods, and overall health. As empaths, this feeling is intensified. We are constantly taking on the energy of others, which can lead to us feeling overwhelmed, drained, and exhausted. If we don't take steps to protect our energy, we can quickly become burned out. As the expression goes, you can't pour from an empty cup. So in order to be there for others, we need to make sure we're taking care of ourselves first. Luckily, there are many ways to heal and protect your energy.

A professional athlete needs to take care of her body so that she can perform at her best. Without the proper nutrition, sleep, rest, and recovery, she won't be able to perform at her highest level. The same is true for us as empaths and intuitives. We need to make sure we're taking care of our bodies, minds, and spirits so that we can show up fully for ourselves and others. Although it's not a competition, think of it as strength and endurance training for the marathon of life.

To help protect our energy, it's important to create boundaries. This means learning to say no when we need to and setting limits with the people in our lives. It also means being mindful of the places we go and the things we do. If we're constantly surrounding ourselves with chaotic energy, it's going to be very difficult to stay grounded and centred. So make sure you're spending time in environments that are peaceful and calming. This could be in nature, a quiet place in your home, or anywhere else that feels safe and serene.

In addition to the basics, such as sleep, nutrition, and exercise, it's important to control our stress levels. Stress can take a toll on our physical and mental health, so it's important to find healthy ways to cope with it. Some people find relief in yoga, meditation, or other forms of relaxation. Others find comfort in journaling, talking to a therapist, or spending time with friends and family. Whatever works for you, make sure you're taking the time to do things that make you feel good and help you relax. Now, let's dive into some specific techniques you can use to heal and protect your energy.

MEDITATION FOR CLEANSING YOUR ENERGY

One of the best ways to protect your energy is through meditation. Meditation helps to quiet the mind and allows us to focus on the present moment. When we're able to be more mindful, we're better able to control our thoughts and emotions. This can be extremely helpful when we're feeling overwhelmed or drained. Meditation helps us to create space between ourselves and the outside world. It allows us to hit the reset button and recharge our batteries. For empaths, meditation can be a lifesaver.

If you're new to meditation, there are many different ways to do it. You don't need to sit for hours in silence or chant mantras. It's important to find a practice that works for you. There are many different approaches, and plenty of free online resources to help you get started. There are also apps, such as Headspace and Calm, that offer guided meditations. Plus, YouTube is full of great meditation videos. You can choose from guided meditations, meditation music, or even simply sitting in silence. Experiment with different types of meditation until you find one that you enjoy. Once you find a style that you like, stick with it and make it a regular part of your routine.

Many newbies are resistant to meditating because they think it's too difficult or time-consuming. But the truth is, anyone can meditate. And it doesn't have to take hours out of your day. Even a few minutes of meditation can make a big difference. Start small and gradually increase the amount of time you spend meditating. Remember, the goal is not to set the Guinness record as the world's longest meditator. The goal is to find some peace and quiet in a world that's constantly trying to grab our attention.

You can begin with five minutes a day and gradually work your way up. You'll be amazed at how much of a difference this simple practice can make. The most important thing is to be consistent and make meditation a part of your daily routine. The more you meditate, the more benefits you'll experience.

USING BREATH TO CHANGE YOUR LIFE

Don't underestimate the healing power of the breath! Breathing exercises are a fantastic way to manage your emotions and protect your energy. When you're stressed, your breathing becomes shallow and erratic. This can lead to feelings of anxiety and panic. By focusing on your breath, you can help to calm the mind and ease these anxious feelings.

In yoga, for example, there is a focus on the breath. This is because the breath is seen as the link between the mind and body. When you control your breath, you're better able to control your thoughts and emotions. And as you already know, our emotional state has a big impact on our energy and our physical body.

Yogic Breath

The yogic breath, also known as ujjayi breath, is a great breathing exercise. To do this exercise, simply inhale and exhale through the nose. As you breathe in, make sure your throat is slightly constricted so that you can hear your breath. Imagine the air passing through your nose and throat as you breathe. This should create a soft 'hissing' sound.

When you're ready, inhale slowly and deeply, filling your lower abdomen first and then letting the breath fill up your mid-torso and upper chest. As you inhale, feel the breath expanding outward in all directions—to the front, to the sides, and to the back. As the breath moves upward, imagine it filling up your whole body with healing energy.

When your abdomen and chest are full of breath, pause for a moment before exhaling. First, release the breath from your upper chest, then from your mid-torso, and finally from your lower abdomen. As you exhale, imagine all the tension and stress leaving your body and dissolving into thin air. After exhaling completely, take a few moments to notice how you feel. Are you more refreshed, awake, and relaxed? Try this exercise for a couple of minutes and see the difference it makes.

This technique is very calming and helps to slow down the breath. It's a great way to ease anxiety and stress. Plus it can be done anywhere and at any time. You don't need any special equipment. Simply focus on your breath and let the rest fall away.

4-7-8 Breath

Another favorite exercise of mine is the 4-7-8 breath exercise, also known as "relaxing breath." To do this exercise, simply breathe in for four counts, hold your breath for seven counts, and then breathe out for eight counts. I like to do it before bed to help me relax and get a restful night's sleep. I've even used it to calm my nerves before delivering an important presentation at work.

By focusing on your breath, you can let go of any racing thoughts and clear your mind. By slowing down and focusing on each breath, you can help to ease anxiety and stress. And by breathing out for a longer count than you breathe in, you can help to calm the nervous system. This exercise is simple, but it can be very effective. Give it a try and see how you feel.

If these breathing exercises seem simple, that's the point. They're meant to be easy to do, so you can easily incorporate them into your daily routine regardless of where you are or what you are doing. Remember, you don't need to contort your body into strange positions or engage in complex spiritual rituals to reap the benefits of breathwork. Simply let the breath be your anchor in the present moment. And let it lead you to a place of peace, calm, and self-control.

By tuning out distractions and connecting with your breath, you will take charge of your energy and your physical body. And when you're in a calm and grounded state of mind, you will enjoy the clarity and focus you need to develop your intuition.

WHITE LIGHT PROTECTION

Visualization is another great way to heal and protect your energy. This exercise involves picturing a white light surrounding your body. This white light is a symbol of protection and love. It helps to keep negative energy out and positive energy in. When you picture this white light around you, visualize it coming down from the sky, enveloping your body, and filling you up with its healing energy, like a big, warm hug.

This exercise is very simple, but it can be extremely powerful. It's a great way to quickly cleanse your energy whenever you're feeling off. You can also use it any time you're around negative people or heavy energy. Simply take a few deep breaths and visualize that bubble of white light surrounding you. This will help to keep you grounded and protected. This bubble is impenetrable and will protect you from any outside negativity like a shield.

I've personally used this exercise on many occasions and felt an instant release. It's a quick and easy way to cleanse your aura and protect yourself from outside forces. You can easily do this while taking public transport, sitting in a coffee shop, or even at your desk at work. It's kind of fun to imagine yourself walking around in a giant white bubble! Plus, it's not like anyone can see what you're doing!

GROUNDING YOUR ENERGY

Taking the time to ground your energy is a great way to keep yourself calm, collected, and centred—especially when things get tough. It is also a great technique to protect yourself from negative energies, both from within and from others. If you're new to this practice, don't worry—it's easy to do.

Simply start by standing on the ground (outside in bare feet is best, but if that's not possible, anywhere is okay). Close your eyes and take a few deep breaths to relax. Now, visualize your body from your head to your toes. Imagine that you are a majestic tree with roots attached to your feet that go deep into the ground. See how these roots grow deeper and deeper into Mother Earth until they reach the center of the planet. Allow yourself to feel how these roots are anchoring you to the ground, making you feel strong, stable, and connected.

Once your roots reach the center of the Earth, visualize how all negative energies within you (fears, energies from others, worries) are transported through your roots to this core. Imagine them being released into the earth, where they dissipate harmlessly and transform into positive, healing energy.

Then envision your body pulling up fresh, clean energy from the Earth to replace the negative energies that have been released. See this energy entering through your roots and filling your entire body with a bright white light.

Allow yourself to feel how this light is cleansing and invigorating your whole being. When you're ready, open your eyes and take a few deep breaths. Notice how calm, centred, and energized you feel. You are strong, stable, and rooted in your truth. You are not swayed by the winds of change or the opinions of others.

SETTING ENERGETIC BOUNDARIES

Personal boundaries are about self-care. They're about giving yourself permission to say "no" to things that don't feel good or that are too much for you. Energetic boundaries are an extension of that. They're about setting limits with other people and situations—drawing a line in the sand and saying "this far, and no further."

We don't get upset with neighbors who put up a fence to mark their property lines, so why is it so difficult for empaths to do the same thing energetically? Well, just like personal boundaries, energetic boundaries are all about self-respect. They help you to protect your energy, your aura, and your space.

Think about it—when you're around someone who is always complaining, it can be exhausting. You might start to feel like you're "absorbing" their energy. Or maybe there's a situation that you keep getting pulled into, even though it doesn't serve you. By setting an energetic boundary, you can remove yourself from that toxic energy and create some space. Energetic boundaries are very practical, and I think everyone can benefit from setting them.

It's also essential to clarify what boundaries are and what they are not. First of all, a boundary is not a wall. A boundary is not about shutting people out or putting up a barrier to keep people away. That's not what boundaries are for. Instead, consider a boundary as a filter. It's a way to let in the good stuff (the energy, the people, the situations) and keep out the bad stuff. Just like a coffee filter, it allows the coffee to flow through, but it catches all the grounds and bits of the coffee beans. You wouldn't want coffee grounds in your cup, right? In the same way, an energetic boundary lets in the good stuff (love, support, positive energy) and keeps out the bad stuff (toxicity, drama, negative energy).

Second, a boundary is not about control. Again, I think this is an important distinction to make. When you set a boundary, you are not trying to control the other person or the situation. Just like you have every right to your physical body, you also have the right to your energetic body. You get to decide who and what you allow into your space. Just because someone else is comfortable with a certain level of drama or toxicity doesn't mean that you have to be. You are simply taking responsibility for yourself and your own energy. Remember—you can't control anyone but yourself. All you can do is set your own limits and stick to them.

Setting boundaries also does not mean that you lack compassion. Many empaths feel guilty about setting boundaries or saying no. Although it's tempting to cheer people up and try to make them feel better, sometimes that's not what others need. Sometimes people need to experience their own emotions and work through their own stuff. And that's okay. It's not your job to make sure everyone is happy all the time. You are allowed to put yourself first, and you are allowed to say no if it means taking care of yourself.

Finally, a boundary is not static. Just like everything else in life, your boundaries will change over time. As you grow and evolve, your needs and relationships will change, and so will your boundaries. What worked for you last year might not work for you now. That's all part of the process. Give yourself permission to change your mind and to change your boundaries as needed.

Techniques to Set Healthy Boundaries

Now that we've got all that straightened out, let's talk about how to set these energetic filters. The first step is to become aware of your own energy. Start paying attention to how you feel around certain people or in certain situations. If you start to feel drained, or if you start to feel like you're being pulled in too deep, that's a sign that you need to set up new boundaries.

The second step is to get clear on what you need. Decide what is acceptable to you and what is not.

What do you need to feel better? Do you need more space? Do you need to take a break from certain people or situations? Once you know what you need, you can figure out solutions that will work for you.

The third step is to take action. It might mean saying no to plans, or it might mean speaking up and asking for what you need. It might even mean ending a relationship—either with a person or with a situation. Whatever it is, stand up for yourself and make sure you follow through.

You might be wondering, *How do I tell someone that I need more space?* There are a few different ways to do this, but I like to keep it simple. I like to use the "sandwich method," which is basically just saying what you need, followed by why, and then ending with a thank you.

For example, let's say you need to take a break from a friend who is always asking for favors. You might say something like this: "Hey, I hope you don't mind if I take a rain check on that coffee date. I've been feeling really overwhelmed lately, and I need some time to myself. Thanks for understanding."

Or let's say you need to set boundaries with your boss, who is always asking you to work overtime. You might say something like this: "I would love to help, but I need to stick to my 9-5 schedule so I have enough time for my other commitments. Thanks for respecting my time." Of course, you can rephrase this however you want, but the important thing is to be clear and direct. The sandwich approach softens the blow and makes it more likely that the other person will be receptive to your request.

Remember, setting boundaries is not about making other people happy—it's about taking care of yourself. So don't be afraid to put yourself first. Your well-being is worth it. It might feel awkward at first, as if you're being rude or ungrateful, but trust me, it gets easier with practice. And people will respect you for it. The more assertive you are, the more likely it is that your boundary will be respected. Your energy is your responsibility. No one else is going to take care of it for you. So make sure you nurture it and protect it so that you can live a happy, healthy, and fulfilling life.

SHIELDING YOUR ENERGY

Energetic boundaries distinguish between what's you and what's not. They are a little bit different from physical boundaries, but the basic principle is the same. You are taking responsibility for your own body, emotions, and your own space, and you are setting limits on what is acceptable.

Energetic boundaries are important because they help you to stay in alignment with your highest self. When you have strong boundaries, you are less likely to get caught up in other people's stuff, and you are more likely to stay focused on your own path.

It's a great practice to "put on your shield" as part of your morning routine. Visualize a protective energetic shield around you when you wake up in the morning or anytime you feel like you need a little extra protection. You can also say an affirmation that resonates with you, such as "I am surrounded by healing light" or "I am safe and protected." This shield is stronger than the most powerful negative force, so you can relax and know that you are safe.

With the energetic armor around you, it is important to also have an open heart. An open heart means that you are willing to receive love and support from the Universe. Trust that the Universe has your back and that you are open to receiving guidance and help when you need it.

When your heart is open, and your boundaries are strong, you are in a great place to create healthy relationships with others and make an impact. You will attract people into your life who respect your boundaries and who are also interested in personal growth. These are the kinds of relationships that nurture and support your soul's evolution.

NATURE HEALS AND RESTORES

There is something special about spending time in nature. The breeze, the trees, the sun and sky...all of it fills us with a sense of peace and restored energy. Being in nature is like a breath of fresh air (pun intended), and it's the perfect way to disconnect from the stressors of our everyday lives. It's no wonder that spending time outdoors has been linked with better mental health!

For highly-sensitive and intuitive empaths, nature is not only a restorative oasis, but also a necessary one. If we don't take time for regular nature breaks, we can easily become bogged down by all the negativity and lose touch with our own positive energy. But nature isn't just good for the soul—it's also good for the physical body. Studies have shown that spending time in nature can lower blood pressure, reduce stress hormone levels, and boost immune function. Being outdoors has also been linked with lower rates of obesity, heart disease, and diabetes.

But I live in a busy city! you might be thinking. *I don't have time to drive out to the woods every weekend.* No problem! Even small doses of nature can have an impact. Something as simple as taking a walk in the park or sitting outside for a few minutes can help you feel more connected to the natural world and balance your energy.

I've experienced the healing power of nature firsthand. Ever since my daughter was born, I've made a conscious effort to go for daily nature walks. It doesn't matter if it's raining or snowing—I bundle up and head out the door. Originally, my motivation was to get her out of the house so she could get some fresh air in the stroller. But I quickly realized that these walks were having a positive effect on my own mental state as well. If I were feeling stressed or overwhelmed, a half-hour spent outdoors would help me to feel more grounded and centred. As a new mom, having that daily nature break became essential for my well-being.

Now, on the rare occasion when I can't go outside, I feel antsy and out of sorts. I've come to rely on my daily nature fix to help me stay balanced and connected. I've also found that the most creative ideas and solutions to problems come to me when I'm outside in nature. There's just something about being in the presence of trees and open space that allows my mind to wander and my inspiration to flow.

If you're an empath, I encourage you to find a way to incorporate regular nature time into your life. It doesn't have to be a big production—a simple walk around the block will do the trick!

Your mind, body, and soul will thank you for it!

SELF-CARE FOR EMPATHS

LET'S GET PHYSICAL!

Taking care of our physical bodies is important for everyone, but it's especially crucial for empaths who tend to be "energy sponges." We tend to feel things more deeply than others, and that can lead to a build-up of stress in the body. Exercise is one of the best ways to release this tension and keep our energy balanced. Exercise helps to get the creative juices flowing by getting the blood pumping to the brain. And when we're physically healthy, we're better able to handle the challenges that come our way—both emotionally and mentally.

There are endless exercise options out there, so you can definitely find something that fits your preferences and lifestyle. Personally, I love dancing and weight training. Moving to music makes me feel joyful and alive. Plus, it's a fun way to bond with my kids. Lifting weights makes me feel like a superhero in training, even when lifting three-pound dumbbells. But there are endless possibilities, so find what you enjoy doing! Exercise doesn't have to be torture —it can (and should!) be something that you look forward to. When it's something you enjoy, you're much more likely to stick with it in the long run. So get out there and move your body!

NOURISHING YOUR BODY

Eating for empaths is not just food. It's fuel for the body, yes, but it's also medicine for the soul. When we put the right foods into our bodies, we feel calmer, more grounded, and more connected to our intuition. But when we eat processed junk food, our brains become scattered, anxious, and disconnected.

Having gone through an emotional rollercoaster with my own diet in my teens and twenties, I can attest to the fact that what we eat makes a big difference in how we feel. I used to survive on a diet of processed foods, caffeine, and sugar. Not surprisingly, it was quite the ride! I felt out of control, anxious, and depressed during my university days. But after making some changes and learning to fuel my body with whole foods, I found that my moods stabilized and my anxiety decreased.

Because we are so connected to the energy of the food we eat, it's important to be mindful of what we put into our bodies. When we eat foods that are heavy in chemicals and pesticides, we're taking in those negative energies as well. Foods that are high in sugar and processed carbohydrates can cause us to feel anxious and irritable, while healthy fats and proteins help us to feel calmer and more grounded.

But when we eat clean, nutritious meals that are nourishing to the body, we feel lighter, brighter, and more aligned with our highest selves. The best diet for empaths is one that is based on fresh, whole foods. This includes plenty of vegetables, fruits, nuts, seeds, and healthy fats. Eating organic whenever possible will also help you avoid exposure to harmful chemicals and pesticides.

Some empaths choose to eat plant-based diets, while others need to have meat or fish in their diet to feel balanced. There are no hard and fast rules here.

Listen to your body and let it guide you to the foods that help you feel your best. Be sure to consult with a healthcare professional before making any major changes to your diet. If you plan on cutting out any food groups, it's important to do so safely with the help of a professional. This is why it's so important for us to eat foods that help us to stay emotionally balanced.

There is no one-size-fits-all approach to nutrition. We are all unique beings with different needs. Some people have sensitivities, others make choices based on ethical reasons, and others have religious or spiritual beliefs that guide their food choices. The most important thing is to be mindful of what you're putting into your body and how it makes you feel. So listen to your body (or your nutritionist!) and let it guide you to the foods that nourish your soul.

WATER IS THE ELIXIR OF LIFE

Water is one of the most powerful elements on Earth. It has the ability to cleanse and purify, and it is essential for life. This is why water is such a powerful tool for detoxing and cleansing the body. If doctors recommend drinking at least eight glasses of water per day, it's mind-boggling that 75 percent of

Americans are chronically dehydrated. We need to remind ourselves to drink water regularly throughout the day, especially when we feel fatigued or stressed.

The truth is that water is essential for our health and well-being. It's involved in every single function of the body, from flushing toxins out of vital organs to keeping the skin clear and hydrated. When we don't drink enough water, our bodies can't function optimally. We may experience fatigue, brain fog, and headaches, among other ailments.

When we drink plenty of water, we are cleansing our bodies of the negative energy that we absorb from others. This helps to keep us grounded and connected to our intuition. When we are hydrated, we are better able to process emotions and stay balanced. Drinking at least eight glasses of water a day is a good way to start. You can also add some fresh lemon juice to your water to help cleanse the liver and promote detoxification. Drinking water seems so basic, but its importance can not be overestimated!

When we submerge ourselves in a body of water, we are entering into a state of purity and stillness. This allows us to clear away any negative energy or emotions that may be clouding our minds and hearts. In this state of stillness, we can access our intuition and connect with our higher selves more easily.

There are many ways to detox with water. You can add some fresh herbs, essential oils, or salts to your bathwater. Celtic sea salt and Himalayan pink salt are both great for detoxing, rejuvenating, and relaxing the body. If you live near a lake or ocean, take some time to swim or meditate by the water's edge. Just being in nature can help to cleanse and purify your energy.

You can also try cold water therapy, which is said to help boost the immune system and promote healthy circulation. My aunt, who lives in Siberia, swears by this method! Siberia is one of the coldest parts of Russia, and she has been doing the polar swim every year to stay healthy. Every winter, she takes a dip in the freezing cold waters of Lake Baikal. A team of brave neighbors dig a hole in the ice, put on their summer swimsuits, and jump right in! To be honest, I get chills just thinking about it. My guess is not everyone reading this book will be willing to freeze their butts off like that, but you can try a cold shower instead.

As you take a refreshing shower, swim in the ocean, or soak in a warm saltwater bath, visualize everything that no longer serves you being washed away. Feel the negativity leaving your body as you surround yourself with the healing power of water. When you're feeling down, stressed out, or just need a break from the world, jump in the shower and let the water wash away your troubles. You'll get an instant boost of energy, and you'll feel refreshed and invigorated.

IMPROVING SLEEP QUALITY

It wasn't until I had kids that I realized how important sleep is. When I was pregnant with my son, other parents used to tell me to get all the sleep I could get before the baby was born. They weren't kidding! Before having kids, I used to stay up late working on my side projects, pull all-nighters watching movies, and I would sleep in until noon on the weekends. I thought I was doing just fine, but then I had babies, and everything changed. I can't recall the last time I had more than three hours of uninterrupted sleep. They're lucky they're that cute! Lack of sleep is no joke. I'm not complaining; I absolutely love being a mom. I am just not a big fan of being a zombie mom. I've had to find ways to function on very little sleep. That, combined with postpregnancy hormones, was not a pretty picture.

Luckily, naps help, and so does a bit of caffeine.

When we don't get enough sleep, our sensitivity to stress increases, and our ability to cope with everyday challenges decreases. We become more irritable, anxious, and moody. Our immune system is also weaker when we're sleep deprived, which means we're more likely to get sick. In order to function at our best and manage our energy, it's important to get enough rest. Unfortunately, for many empaths, getting proper sleep can be a challenge. We tend to absorb other people's energy, which can keep us up at night.

> *"I can't turn off my thoughts. My mind just keeps racing from all the energy I picked up during the day."*
>
> *"I tend to have nightmares or very vivid dreams that leave me feeling drained and exhausted when I wake up."*
>
> *"I comfort myself with food when I'm feeling sleep-deprived, overwhelmed, or stressed."*

If you can relate to these confessions from other empaths, then it's time to prioritize your sleep. Start by setting the intention that you will have a restful sleep. Then do something calming such as reading, meditating, or taking a bath. It's also helpful to write down any thoughts or worries that are on your mind so you can release them before going to bed.

It's also recommended to avoid using electronic devices in the hours leading up to sleep, as the blue light emitted can disrupt your body's natural sleep cycle. Another helpful tip is to avoid caffeine in the afternoon and evening, as it can stay in your system for 6-8 hours. You can replace it with herbal tea or decaffeinated coffee. And don't forget the meditation and grounding exercises can be very helpful in calming the mind and body before sleep. We need sleep for our physical and mental health, so make it a priority.

THE MAGIC POWER OF CRYSTALS

As an empath, I can feel when someone is having a bad day or is carrying around negative energy. It can be overwhelming at times, and I have to be very careful about who I let into my personal space. One of the best ways to protect your energy is by wearing gemstone jewelry. Gemstones are powerful stones that can help to deflect bad vibes and throw up a forcefield around you.

When I wear my gemstone necklace, I feel like I have a layer of protection around me that helps me to stay grounded and safe. Healing crystals can be worn as jewelry, carried in your pocket, or placed around your home. It might just be the thing that helps you to feel more balanced and in control.

Let's explore some of the most popular crystals for empaths, their healing properties, and how they can benefit you!

Rose Quartz

When it comes to protection, empaths often think they need to build walls in order to keep themselves safe. However, this doesn't have to be the case. There are other ways to protect yourself, and one of them is by using the rose quartz stone. The rose quartz is a heart chakra stone that promotes peace, inner harmony, and positive energy. It can help you stay soaked in the light of love, even when the darkest moods try to bring the clouds.

Additionally, rose quartz washes away toxic emotions and purifies bad air. So if you're holding on to bad energy, this soft pink stone can quickly cleanse it away. This makes rose quartz a powerful tool for protection, helping you to keep your energy positive and negativity at bay.

Amethyst

Amethyst is a beautiful purple gemstone that has been used for centuries for its mystical properties. According to ancient lore, amethyst is a powerful talisman that can protect against psychic attacks and nurture one's own psychic abilities. Amethyst is also said to be helpful in promoting sweet sleep, easing anxieties, and removing negative or toxic energies. In addition to its many metaphysical properties, amethyst is also simply lovely to look at—no wonder it is such a popular gemstone! Whether you are drawn to amethyst for its beauty or its healing powers, this gemstone is sure to bring you some peace and relaxation.

Aventurine

Aventurine is a powerful stone that is said to bring good luck and fortune. It is also known for its ability to help heal emotional wounds and traumas. If you are facing a challenging situation or a major life change, aventurine can help you to overcome any obstacles in your way. It is also said to promote creativity, self-confidence, and inner strength. To get the most out of this healing stone, sit quietly with it for a while and let its light and energy work their magic. You may just find the courage and strength you need to overcome whatever challenges come your way.

Lapis Lazuli

In today's fast-paced world, it can be easy to get caught up in the opinions of others and lose sight of our own inner wisdom. Lapis lazuli is a powerful stone that helps us to stay tuned in to our own intuition and find the courage to speak our truth. This beautiful blue stone has been used since ancient times to open the third eye chakra and connect us with higher realms of consciousness. It helps us to see beyond the veils of illusion and tap into our own inner knowing.

When we wear or carry lapis, we are reminded to stay true to ourselves and follow our own unique path in life, even when it isn't the popular opinion. This is a stone of self-empowerment that grants us the strength to stand up for what we believe in and express our authentic selves. Whether you are an empath who is easily affected by others' energy, or you simply need a reminder to stay connected to your own inner guidance, lapis lazuli is the perfect stone for you.

Agate

Brown agate is a stabilizing and grounding stone that helps keep you rooted even when emotional turbulence is high. It has the ability to create a shield against negative energy, and rather than just blocking it, brown agate bounces back bad energy and transforms it into something positive. This makes it an incredibly powerful ally for those who are seeking emotional balance and protection from negativity. In addition to its defensive capabilities, brown agate is also a very comforting stone that connects you to the earthy energies of nature, promoting stability and calm. If you are looking for a stone that can help you weather life's storms, brown agate is a great choice.

Hematite

Hematite is a strong, powerful stone with a deep meaning. It is known as the warrior stone, and for good reason—hematite helps us to tap into our own sense of survival and intuition. It can teach us how to protect ourselves from unwanted energies and how to compartmentalize the energies of others so that we don't become overwhelmed. Hematite has a silvery black sheen that is both beautiful and sleek, making it the perfect stone to wear as a protective shield. When we work with hematite, we are reminded of our own strength and courage—two things that we need in order to stand tall and proud. If you're looking for a stone that will help you feel more confident and empowered, then hematite is definitely one to consider.

Moonstone

Moonstone is a beautiful, milky white stone that is said to be laced with feminine energy. It is known as a healing crystal that can chase away the shadows. It is also known as the stone of the mother moon. Moonstone is said to be a traveller's stone, keeping all those safe out on the road. For sensitive souls, moonstone can enhance intuition and bring about good fortune. It is also said to keep bad energy at bay and ensure that you stay linked to the light of the divine. Moonstone is definitely a stone worth learning more about!

Clear Quartz

Clear quartz opens the mind and heart to higher guidance, amplifying your thoughts and prayers. It filters out distractions, providing clarity for those who want to move forward in life with a more positive outlook. Clear quartz crystal is also known as the master healer, making it an excellent choice for empaths who are looking for an emotional balancing stone. When combined with other crystals, the clear quartz amplifies their effects and makes them even more powerful. So if you're looking for a crystal that can help bring calmness, emotional balance, and clarity into your life, clear quartz is a great choice.

Malachite

Malachite is a beautiful green mineral that has many different uses. It is most commonly used in jewelry and ornamental objects, but it can also be used for its energetic properties. Malachite is said to shift stagnant energies and bring freshness to the air around you. It is also a heart chakra stone that builds trust and love and encourages positive change. Malachite is a great stone for empaths as it helps with building resilience and inner wisdom. It also helps to keep the flow of energy running clear from tip to toe. In addition, it can assist you with personal growth and transformation!

Citrine

Citrine is a stone that is often associated with the sun and its radiant energy. The name citrine comes from the French word "citron," meaning lemon. It is also sometimes called "success stone" or "merchant's stone." Citrine is said to promote and manifest success and abundance, especially in business. It is also used to increase self-confidence, personal power, and will. Citrine is a solar plexus chakra stone that helps you to harness your personal power and increase your confidence to go after your dreams. When your solar plexus chakra is in balance, you feel calm, confident, and in control of your life. Citrine can also help to clear out any blockages or negative energies that are holding you back from reaching your full potential. If you are looking for a stone that will help you to manifest your desires and boost your creative spirit, citrine is a great option for you.

Amazonite

Amazonite is a stunning blue-green stone that has long been associated with the ancient Amazon warriors of South America. According to legend, these fierce women used amazonite as a talisman to protect themselves from harm in battle. Today, amazonite is still revered as a powerful stone of protection, but it is also prized for its ability to promote intuition, emotional intelligence, and proactive thinking. If you are seeking clarity and guidance, amazonite can help you to tap into your inner wisdom and find your true path.

This stone is also excellent for those who are looking to build healthy boundaries in their relationships. By aligning your personal values with your intuition, amazonite can help you to create relationships that are based on respect and authenticity. Whether you are looking for protection, guidance, or healthy boundary-setting, amazonite is a forcefield when it comes to tapping into intellect and intuition.

Lepidolite

Lepidolite is a stone that is full of feel-good vibes and is known as the peace stone. This stone is amazing at helping to heal those who feel like they are in emotional overdrive. Whenever you feel the weight of overwhelm, lepidolite can lend a hand to get you back on track. Lepidolite is also very helpful in reducing the impact of electric and magnetic fields (EMFs). In addition, lepidolite clears the gateways that connect the heart, the third eye, and the crown chakra. If you'd like a stone that can help you achieve emotional balance, lepidolite would be a great choice.

Fluorite

Fluorite is a breathtaking stone that shimmers in rainbow shades. It is known for its ability to tap into lower energies and help us feel grounded and strong. Fluorite also helps to clear and heal the third eye chakra. When our root chakra is connected with our third eye chakra, we feel safe and secure. This sense of security is essential for empaths who often need to go with the flow without losing their footing. Fluorite is a powerful stone that can help us to feel balanced and grounded.

Obsidian

There is a lot of power in intuition. It is often our first sense of what is true for us before the mind has a chance to catch up and rationalize it away. But sometimes, we can be afraid to follow our intuition because we don't feel prepared for what it might show us. This is where obsidian can be helpful. Obsidian is a stone that provides protection from negative vibes and toxic thoughts. It can help boost your sense of safety so that you feel free to dive deep into your intuition without being overwhelmed.

When you are able to explore your intuition without fear, you may be surprised at how much wisdom and guidance it has to offer. So if you are feeling like you are holding yourself back or shying away from your sense of truth, reach for some obsidian and see what comes through.

Labradorite

One of my personal favourites, labradorite, is a beautiful gemstone that is said to have mystical qualities. It is believed to help illuminate your intuition and give you the tools you need to explore your destiny. This gemstone is all about discovery and helping you play with possibility. If you are feeling in an energetic slump or unsure of which path to walk, labradorite can help lead the way. You can carry it with you as an amulet or use it as a visualization tool. Labradorite is a powerful gemstone that can help you on your journey of self-discovery.

As you can see, there are many different crystals and stones that can be helpful for empaths to have in their arsenal. Each one offers different benefits that can help you feel more balanced, grounded, and connected. So if you are feeling called to work with crystals, don't be afraid to experiment and see which ones resonate with you. Let your intuition be your guide.

ESSENTIAL OILS TO RAISE YOUR VIBRATION

As an empath, it is essential to have a toolkit of selfcare items to help you navigate through life. Essential oils are powerful plant extracts that can be used to support your health and well-being. They are particularly valuable for chakra healing and balancing.

The skin is the largest organ in the human body. It protects us from the outside world and helps regulate our internal temperature. Our skin also absorbs a lot of what we put on it, including chemicals found in many personal care products. Essential oils are a natural alternative to these products, and they can offer a wide range of benefits. Unlike synthetic chemicals, essential oils work with our body's own systems to promote health and healing. They are increasingly being used in a variety of settings, from spas and salons to hospitals and medical clinics. They're easily accessible and relatively inexpensive, making them a great choice for self-care for empaths.

For example, essential oils can also be used to calm the mind, promote relaxation, enhance psychic abilities, and shield from negative energy. When absorbed through the skin and into the bloodstream, they provide a direct pathway for healing to take place. As their benefits are becoming more widely known, essential oils are becoming a popular choice for self-care.

There are many different ways to use essential oils. You can add them to your bathwater, diffuse them in your home, or apply them directly to your skin.

Not all essential oils are created equal, so be sure to do your research and buy from a reputable source. And always remember to use caution when working with any new substance, including essential oils. Start slowly and pay attention to how your body responds.

And now, I'd like to share with you some of my favorite essential oils for empaths.

Ready, Set an Intention, Go!

Setting an intention is key to unlocking the full power of aromatherapy. When you take the time to focus on why you want to develop your psychic abilities, you open yourself up to receiving all that your chosen essential oil has to offer. Whether you're looking for guidance, clarity, or simply want to connect with your intuition on a deeper level, setting a strong intention will help you to get the most out of your experience. Choose an oil that resonates with your intention, and let the powerful scent work its magic. With a little practice, you'll be surprised at just how intuitively attuned you can become.

Your psychic ability is like a muscle that you need to flex and strengthen in order to develop it. Just like any skill, the more you practice using your intuition, the stronger it will become. But before you can start flexing your "psychic muscles," you need to get clear on your intention. What do you want to achieve? Do you want to develop your ability to read energy? To connect with your spirit guides? To shield yourself from negative energy? Once you have a clear intention, choose an oil that will support your goals.

Some of my favorite oils for psychic development are:

Lavender: Calm and Prevent Anxiety

Lavender has a sweet, floral aroma that is instantly recognizable, and it's no surprise that this oil has been used for centuries in a variety of ways. The Egyptians and Romans used it for bathing, relaxation, cooking, and as perfume.

The soothing aroma of lavender oil has been researched and shown to provide a calming effect on your nervous system and mental state. Many people use lavender oil to remove negative & anxious feelings that prevent them from getting a good night's sleep, too. That being said, being well-rested and calm can help you start your day with positive energy. If you're feeling anxious, give lavender oil a try. You might just be surprised by how much it helps.

You can add it to your bath water to soak away stress or apply it to the temples and the back of the neck. Add a few drops of lavender oil to pillows, bedding, or bottoms of feet to relax and prepare for a restful night's sleep.

Peppermint: Combat Negative Energy

If you're feeling weighed down by negative energy, it might be time to reach for the peppermint oil. Studies have found that peppermint oil aromatherapy could help to reduce feelings of pain and anxiety. Participants reported feeling more relaxed after inhaling the minty scent, and researchers believe that the oil's ability to improve mood and relieve tension could also help to promote mental clarity.

So next time you're feeling stressed or overwhelmed, try diffusing some peppermint oil or dabbing a bit on your temples—you may just find that it helps to clear your mind and give you a much-needed sense of refreshment.

Sweet Orange: Add Some Zest to Your Day

Sweet orange essential oil has been researched over the years and shown to provide a wide variety of positive benefits. One notable advantage that can translate to warding off negative energy is reducing symptoms of depression.

We all know how it feels to be bogged down by stress and sadness when you have a lot on your plate. Thankfully, there is a natural solution that has been proven to help. Sweet orange oil has been shown in multiple studies to reduce stress levels and depressive behaviors. So the next time you are feeling down, reach for the orange oil instead of unhealthy comfort foods. Inhaling the citrusy scent or applying it topically can help to improve your mood and uplift your spirits.

Clary Sage: Develop Your Intuition

Clary sage is an incredible oil that can help us to connect to our third eye. It has a long history of being used spiritually, and it is said to lift the darkness and help us through emotional crises. Clary sage oil is often used in meditation and prayer, as it is said to promote feelings of peace and calm. For empaths and highly sensitive people, clary sage oil can be a valuable ally, helping to ground and protect us from taking on too much negative energy.

Clary sage can also bring clarity, discernment, and expansion. If you are interested in trying it, be sure to get the purest oil you can find. Also, do your research and follow all safety guidelines. When used properly, clary sage can be a powerful tool for spiritual growth.

Lemon Oil: Let's Get Refreshed

Lemon oil is a popular choice for many purposes because it is so versatile. It has a fresh, citrus scent that can promote an open and awake mind—perfect for psychic development! In addition to its psychic benefits, lemon oil can also be used to cleanse and purify your space, as well as to uplift your mood, and boost your energy levels.

Lemon oil is a powerful defender against negative energy and can also be used to cleanse your aura. When added to a diffuser blend, lemon oil can help you to focus and concentrate. It is also said to be helpful in relieving stress and anxiety. Whether you are using it for psychic development or simply to enjoy its refreshing scent, lemon oil is versatile and useful to have on hand.

Tea Tree Oil: Cleanse and Purify Your Space

If you're looking to cleanse your home or workspace of negative energy, tea tree oil is a great choice. This essential oil has long been used in traditional medicine for its cleansing properties, and it can be just as effective at cleansing your environment.

Tea tree oil has natural antibacterial, antiviral, and antifungal properties, making it ideal for purifying your space. It can also help to boost your immune system, which is an important part of protecting yourself from negative energy. To use tea tree oil for cleansing, add a few drops to a diffuser or spray bottle filled with water. You can also add it to a cloth and wipe down surfaces in your home or workspace.

Bergamot: Fight off Fatigue

We all have those days where we just can't seem to shake that tired feeling. No matter how much caffeine we drink or how many naps we take, the fatigue just won't budge. And when we're feeling drained like this, it's often hard to muster up the energy to do the things we need to do.

Using bergamot oil can help reduce feelings of fatigue, making it a great natural remedy for when you're feeling sluggish. So next time you're struggling to get going, reach for the bergamot oil and take a deep breath. You may just find that it's the pick-me-up you need to get back on track.

Rose Oil: Soothe Your Senses

I absolutely adore rose oil! It's one of my all-time favorite essential oils. Not only does it smell divine, but it also has some amazing benefits. Rose oil is said to increase inner harmony and self-love, as well as improve our connection to our higher selves. It's also said to be helpful in times of grief and heartache. I like to use rose oil when I'm meditating or doing energy work. I add a few drops to my diffuser or apply it directly to my skin. If you've never tried rose oil, I highly recommend it!

Cedarwood: Clear the Mind Clutter

As any gifted individual knows, having a clear mind is essential for developing your gifts. Unfortunately, it can be all too easy to get caught up in the day-today clutter of life and lose sight of what's important. That's where cedarwood oil comes in. Cedarwood oil has been used for centuries as a way to promote clarity and focus. It helps to clear away the mental clutter and allows you to focus on your gifts. In addition, it has a calming effect that can help to reduce stress and anxiety. If you're looking for a way to gain ultimate clarity, cedarwood oil is definitely worth trying.

Chamomile: Unwind and Relax

Chamomile is an incredibly versatile and calming oil, making it perfect for diffusing when working on your psychic development. When we allow ourselves to release fears and open our minds to the truth, we create space for real progress. Chamomile can help with this process by reducing stress and anxiety, promoting relaxation, and encouraging feelings of well-being.

Additionally, its soothing aroma can help to ease headaches and promote a good night's sleep. Whether you're just starting out on your psychic development journey or you've been working on it for a while, consider diffusing chamomile oil to help support your practice.

Jasmine: Your Meditation Buddy

Do you love the smell of jasmine? If so, you're in for a treat because this essential oil not only smells fantastic, but it can also be a great meditation buddy. Jasmine has long been used in aromatherapy to promote relaxation and sleep, making it the perfect oil to use before meditating. But that's not all—jasmine can also help increase psychic dreams! So if you meditate at night, use jasmine in your diffuser, have your dream journal handy and get ready to receive intuitive messages while you sleep.

Geranium Rose: Get Connected

Geranium rose is a beautiful smelling oil that helps to raise your vibration. I like to use it before meditation, as it allows me to connect more easily with my guides and angels. Simply rub a few drops in your palms and inhale deeply a few times. This will help you to relax and receive messages more easily. You can also use it on your third eye for deeper meditation and visioning. It smells amazing and will help you to feel more connected and at ease.

Frankincense: The King of Oils

There's a reason why frankincense is often referred to as the "king of oils." Frankincense is one of my favorite oils because it has such a high vibration. It's like having a little magic in a bottle that you can use to uplift your mood and protect yourself spiritually. I like to apply it to the back of my neck or use a diffuser with a few drops. You can also apply it to a scarf or diffuser necklace so you can smell it throughout the day. If you're feeling exhausted from being around people, massage some frankincense over your heart chakra and ask your guides to surround you with love and protect you from negativity. It's an amazing oil that I always keep in my collection.

Sandalwood: Enjoy Your Sacred Space

Sandalwood has been used for centuries in meditation and prayer. The wood has a deep, earthy scent that is said to open the soul and promote healing. Although sandalwood is woody and dry, it is also very fragrant. This essential oil helps to focus the mind and can be used in meditation to promote spiritual awakening. The scent of sandalwood is said to bring us into a state of receptivity, which can be helpful when we are seeking guidance or healing. If you are curious about how sandalwood can help you on your spiritual journey, consider using it in your next meditation or prayer practice.

Whether you're just getting started on your journey with aromatherapy or you've been using essential oils for a while, these oils can help to support your practice. By diffusing or applying them before meditation, you can shield yourself from negative energy, increase your vibration, and connect more easily with your intuition. They are like a bridge that helps us to connect with the spiritual realm. When we use them in meditation or prayer, we create a sacred space that allows us to receive guidance and healing. The oils help to open our minds and hearts, and their aromatic scents guide us on our journey.

CREATE A SANCTUARY THAT SUPPORTS YOU

As an empath, I know how important it is to have a safe place to retreat to when the world feels overwhelming. Having a personal sanctuary gives you a place to recharge and recalibrate your energy. It's important to have a space that is just for you, where you can go to relax and feel at peace. I like to call it a "sanctuary," but really, it can be any place that brings you comfort and peace. A bedroom, a corner in your living room, or even a spot in nature where you can go to connect with yourself.

Creating a sanctuary is all about having an environment that supports you. It doesn't have to be complex or fancy. The most important thing is that it feels safe and nurturing to you. I'll give you some ideas of things you can do to create a sanctuary, but it really comes down to what feels right for you.

Let's dive in!

Declutter

One of the most important things you can do to create a sanctuary is to clear the space. This means getting rid of anything that doesn't support your ability to relax and feel at ease. If you're not sure where to start, consider doing a quick sweep of the room and getting rid of anything that doesn't bring you joy.

This could be anything from old books that you no longer need, clothes on your floor, or decorations on the shelves that no longer serve a purpose. Personally, I find my level of anxiety goes up when my space gets messy or cluttered, so I make it a point to declutter on a regular basis. Even if it's just a few minutes a day, decluttering and organizing can make a big difference in how you feel. Since even things have energy, it's important to surround yourself with things that make you feel good.

If you're unsure where to start, I recommend checking out the book *The Life-Changing Magic of Tidying Up* by Marie Kondo. It's a great resource for decluttering your space and only keeping things that bring you joy.

The KonMari method described in the book involves going through your belongings one by one and deciding whether or not to keep them. It's simple: If it doesn't spark joy, then you get rid of it. Of course, this might sound easier said than done because most people tend to hang on to things for sentimental reasons. However, if you're really honest with yourself about what brings you happiness, you might be surprised at how little you actually need to keep.

I feel like a new person when my surroundings are clean and clutter-free. It's as if the physical act of decluttering also clears out my mind. In return, this allows me to feel more relaxed and at ease in my home. Many spiritual teachers also assert that decluttering creates more space for abundance in your life. When you let go of what no longer serves you, you make room for new and better things to come into your life. I couldn't agree more.

Sage Your Space

Once you've cleared the physical space, it's time to focus on the energetics of the space.

Sage is an amazing tool for clearing energy. It's been used for centuries in many different cultures. If you're new to saging, the basic idea is that you burn sage and let the smoke waft through your space. As the smoke clears, it also removes any negative energy from the space.

It's good practice to sage your space regularly, especially if you live in a city or have a lot of people coming in and out of your home. I like to sage my space at least once a week, but you can do it whenever you have a feeling like you need to reset the energy.

The first time I saw someone sage a space, I was a bit sceptical. I mean, how could smoke have clear energy? But I decided to give it a try, and I was surprised at how effective it was. Not only did my space feel energetically lighter, but I also felt more peaceful and at ease.

If you're interested in trying it out, you can buy sage online or at most health food stores. There are also smudge sticks available that you can burn. I personally like to use loose sage because I find it easier to control the smoke.

To sage your space, open all of the doors and windows in the room. Then light the sage and let the smoke waft through the space. You can use your hand to help direct the smoke into all of the corners and nooks of the room. As you do this, say a prayer or affirmation such as "I release all negative energy from this space." You can also sage yourself by wafting the smoke around your body. When you're finished, be sure to open the doors and windows to let the smoke out.

This is a simple yet effective way to create a more positive and peaceful home. By taking the time to do this on a regular basis, you can create an environment that supports your well-being and allows you to thrive.

Bring in Some Nature

Plants are a great way to purify the air and add some life to your space. Energetically, they help to raise the vibration of your space and create a more positive environment. They also help to filter out toxins from the air, which is especially important if you live in a city.

Plants such as aloe vera, snake plant, and Boston fern are all great options for purifying the air. If you don't have a green thumb, cacti and succulents are also great options because they don't require a lot of water or maintenance.

I'm a big fan of greenery in the house, so my philosophy about plants is similar to my philosophy about art. I believe that you should surround yourself with things that make you happy. So if plants make you happy, then, by all means, fill your space with them!

Every time I walk into a room and see a plant, it makes me think of a lush oasis. There are many different ways to incorporate plants into your home. You can put them in pots and place them around the room, or you can create a living wall by hanging plants from a rack. You can also make your own terrariums or buy them online. No matter how you choose to incorporate plants into your space, they will help to create a more positive and peaceful environment.

If you have pets, be sure to do your research before adding plants to your home. Some plants are toxic to animals, so it's important to choose ones that are safe for your furry friends or out of reach.

MAKE A VISION BOARD THAT WORKS

A vision board is a powerful tool that can help you manifest your dreams and goals. The idea is that you create a board with images and words that represent what you want to achieve in your life. This could be anything from a new job or promotion to a trip you want to take or a relationship you want to be in.

Since this book is focused on empathy and developing psychic ability, I would suggest adding images and words that represent these things as well. For example, you could add an image of a person meditating with a shield of protective white light around them or a photo of a person surrounded by butterflies (which are often associated with psychic ability). You could also add words like "intuition," "love," and "healing" or affirmations such as "I trust my intuition," "I am surrounded by love and light," or "I am a powerful healer."

The key is to make your vision board as specific as possible. The more detailed it is, the better. Once you have your vision board created, put it somewhere where you will see it every day. I keep mine in my "personal sanctuary" which is a small space in my home that is just for me. Seeing it every day helps to keep my goals and intentions at the forefront of my mind.

Creating a vision board is not enough on its own to manifest your dreams and goals. You also need to take action steps toward achieving them. But having a visual representation of what you want to achieve can help to keep you motivated and focused on your goals. The KEY is to feel into the energy of what you want to achieve as if it has already happened. So if you want a new job, feel the energy of already having that job. If you want to travel to a specific place, feel the energy of already being there. This is how you attract your goals and dreams into your life. It's not about the board itself but about your emotions. If you can visualize it and feel the emotions of already having it, you will be well on your way to achieving it.

It might sound a bit woo-woo, but trust me, it works like magic! I could write a whole book on the number of goals and dreams I have manifested using this method (and maybe I will one day!). The reason it works is because of the Law of Attraction. This is the universal law that states that like attracts like. So if you are vibrating at a high frequency (which you will be if you are feeling into the energy of already having your goal), then you will attract things of a similar frequency into your life.

Your vision board should make you feel excited, happy, and hopeful about achieving your goals. This is your personal vision board, so there are no rules about what you should or shouldn't include. Make it as creative and fun as you like! And once you tap into the emotions of manifesting your goals, you will be amazed at how quickly they start to show up in physical reality.

BALANCING YOUR CHAKRAS

As a society, we've become pretty obsessed with being healthy. And rightfully so! We only get one body to last us our lifetime, so we might as well take care of it. But when it comes to health, we often focus on the physical aspects and neglect the mental and spiritual. Since we are energetic beings, it's important to pay attention to all three aspects of our health.

And that's where the chakras come in. In Sanskrit, "chakra" means "wheel" or "disk," and they refer to the seven main energy centers in the body. They start at the base of the spine and go all the way up to the crown of the head. Each chakra is associated with different physical, mental, and emotional qualities.

When they're balanced, we feel healthy and whole. Our energy can flow freely, and we feel grounded, connected, creative, confident, and at peace. We are able to give and receive love easily. We feel connected to our higher selves and the universe. We are in alignment with our truth. On the other hand, when our chakras are underactive or overactive, we can feel physical, mental, and emotional distress. This can manifest as anxiety, depression, chronic illnesses, and issues with our relationships.

I'm going to walk you through each chakra and give you some tips on how to keep them balanced. Remember, it's important to listen to your intuition and use whatever resonates with you.

EXPLORING THE 7 CHAKRAS

You can think of chakras as storehouses of energy, each one associated with different areas of your life. By understanding and working with these energies, you can start to create more balance in your life—physically, emotionally, mentally, and spiritually.

If you imagine each chakra as a spinning wheel of energy, they are all interconnected and spin at different speeds. When one chakra is out of balance, it will impact the others. For example, if your root chakra is out of balance, you may feel ungrounded and disconnected from your body. If your solar plexus chakra is out of balance, you may feel insecure or lacking in confidence. Chakra healing is the process of bringing these energies back into alignment so that you can live a more balanced, healthy, and happy life.

There are seven main chakras, each one located at a different point along the spine: the root chakra, sacral chakra, solar plexus chakra, heart chakra, throat chakra, third eye chakra, and the crown chakra. Each one plays a role in our overall health and wellbeing.

There is also a direct connection between chakras and psychic abilities. When the third eye chakra is open and balanced, for example, you're more likely to experience psychic visions and intuitive insights. If you're interested in opening up your intuitive abilities, balancing and healing your chakras is a good place to start.

Root Chakra

The first chakra is the root chakra. It's located at the base of the spine, and it's responsible for our feeling of safety and security. When it's in balance, we feel grounded and stable. For example, we might have a strong sense of our identity and feel confident in who we are. We're able to take care of our basic needs, and we don't feel like life is constantly up in the air.

When the root chakra is out of balance, we can feel insecure, anxious, and disconnected from our bodies. We might feel like we're constantly struggling to make ends meet. We might feel like our lives are out of control. In our fast-paced world, it's easy for the root chakra to become unbalanced.

The color associated with the root chakra is red, and its element is earth. To heal the root chakra, it's important to connect with the physical world and your body. Spend time in nature, eat healthy food, exercise, and get enough sleep. Wear red clothing or jewelry, eat root vegetables, and use red stones like garnet, bloodstone, or black tourmaline. When you focus on balancing the root chakra, you create a foundation of security and confidence that will support you in all areas of your life.

Sacral Chakra

The second chakra is the sacral chakra. It's located just below the navel in the lower abdomen, and it's responsible for our creativity, passion, and sexual energy. When it's in balance, we feel creative, sensual, and confident. We're able to flow with change easily and enjoy our bodies. If you ever feel "in the flow" or like everything is just clicking, it's probably because your sacral chakra is balanced.

When the sacral chakra is out of balance, we can feel creatively blocked, sexually repressed, or emotionally unstable. We might feel like we're stuck in a rut or that our lives are lacking passion. It can also manifest as problems with our reproductive organs, urinary tract infections, sexual dysfunction, or lower back pain. Emotionally, we might feel like we're carrying around a lot of resentment or bitterness.

The sacral chakra is represented by the color orange, and its element is water. To balance and heal the sacral chakra, it's recommended to spend time in water, either by swimming, boating, or simply taking a bath. Wear orange clothing or jewelry, and eat oranges, tangerines, and other citrus fruits. Use orange stones like carnelian, citrine, or coral. Take time to indulge in creative activities and allow yourself to feel your emotions fully. When you focus on balancing the sacral chakra, you create more passion, creativity, and pleasure in your life.

Solar Plexus Chakra

The third chakra is the solar plexus chakra. It's located in the upper abdomen just below the sternum, and it's responsible for our personal power and sense of self-worth. When you see someone who's confident, and in control, they likely have a strong solar plexus chakra.

If your solar plexus chakra is imbalanced, you may feel like you're not good enough or that you don't have what it takes to succeed. You might be easily manipulated by others or find yourself in codependent relationships. When it's out of balance, we can feel powerless and like a victim. We might have digestive issues like ulcers, heartburn, or indigestion. We may also have eating disorders or trouble asserting ourselves.

To heal your solar plexus chakra, try meditating on the color yellow. I like to visualize a bright sun glowing in my belly and filling my whole being with its warm, nourishing energy. You can also try eating yellow foods like lemon, pineapple, and squash or wearing yellow clothing. And don't forget to nourish yourself with healthy food and plenty of self-care!

A balanced solar plexus chakra will help you set healthy boundaries and stand up for yourself. This is essential for empaths who tend to absorb other people's energy. When your solar plexus chakra is balanced, you'll feel confident and in control of your life. You'll know your worth, and you won't let anyone take advantage of you.

You can also try yoga poses that open up the solar plexus area like Cobra Pose or Upward Dog Pose. And finally, essential oils like lemon and ginger can be helpful in balancing this chakra. So give some of these a try and see what works for you!

Heart Chakra

The fourth chakra is the heart chakra. It's located in the center of the chest, and it governs our ability to give and receive love. When it's in balance, we feel open, loving, and compassionate. Empaths tend to have a very strong heart chakra because they are naturally giving and caring people.

If your heart chakra is imbalanced, you may find yourself feeling closed off, resentful, or jealous. You might have a hard time forgiving others or yourself. You may also experience physical symptoms like chest pain, high blood pressure, or difficulty breathing.

To heal your heart chakra, start by meditating on the color green. Visualize a beautiful green healing light emanating from your heart and filling your entire body with its peaceful energy. You can also try eating green foods like kale, spinach, and parsley or wearing green clothing.

Balancing the heart chakra helps us to have healthy relationships with others. We're also able to forgive easily and let go of grudges. When we have a blockage in our heart chakra, we may find it difficult to trust others or open up to them. We may also have a hard time forgiving. This can lead to feelings of loneliness, isolation, and insecurity. We might also put others' needs before our own or find it difficult to set boundaries.

If you suspect you have a blockage in your heart chakra, there are several things you can do to help heal it. First, try to become more aware of your thoughts and emotions. Pay attention to when you're feeling closed off or resistant to love. When you catch yourself thinking negative thoughts about yourself or others, stop and take a few deep breaths. Then try to replace those thoughts with more positive ones.

Throat Chakra

The fifth chakra is the throat chakra. It's located in the center of the throat, and it governs our ability to communicate and express ourselves clearly and confidently. We also have good boundaries and know when to speak up and when to stay silent.

A close friend of mine was going through a challenging time in her marriage, so she went to see a psychic to get some guidance. He noticed that she kept touching her neck and told her that her throat chakra was out of balance and that she needed to start speaking her truth. At first, my friend was resistant. She didn't want to rock the boat or make things worse by speaking up. But the more she thought about it, the more she realized that the intuitive was right. She had been holding back her true feelings for far too long, and it was time to speak up to her husband. She was feeling tired and needed her husband to step in more and help with the kids. She also wanted him to be more attentive and affectionate. So she took a deep breath and had a heart-toheart talk with him. It wasn't easy, but it was so worth it. After that conversation, her relationship improved significantly.

If you're having trouble communicating your needs or speaking your truth, it's likely that your throat chakra is out of balance. You might also find yourself being overly critical of others or yourself. You may find yourself feeling shy, withdrawn, or unable to express yourself. You may also experience physical symptoms like a sore throat, neck pain, or headaches.

There are several things you can do to help balance your throat chakra. One is to meditate on the color blue. Visualize a peaceful blue light filling your throat and spreading to your entire body with its calming energy.

Another way to balance your throat chakra is to simply start speaking your truth. This can be difficult, but it's so important. When you're honest with yourself and others, you open up the channels of communication and allow for more open and honest relationships. You may also want to try journaling or writing down your thoughts and feelings. This can be a great way to release any pent-up emotions and get them out of your system.

Third Eye Chakra

The sixth chakra is the third eye chakra. It's based in the center of the forehead, just above the eyebrows. It governs our ability to see clearly, both physically and intuitively. We also have good concentration, focus, and memory.

I find that when my third eye chakra is in balance, I can think clearly and make good decisions. I'm also able to see things from different perspectives and have a more open mind. Also, looking back, I can see how unbalanced my third eye chakra was when I was younger.

For example, when I was in college, I had a boyfriend who was emotionally abusive. I stayed with him for far too long because I couldn't see the situation clearly. I was so blinded by my love for him that I couldn't see that he was manipulating and controlling me. It wasn't until I finally ended the relationship and got some distance from him that I could see things more clearly. As I became more aware of my own worth, I realized that I deserved so much better. I know that a lot of women and men reading this book will be able to relate to this example.

As empaths, you are blessed with the ability to see and feel things that other people can't. But this gift can also be a curse if you're not careful. You may find yourself being drawn to unhealthy relationships or situations because you can't see them clearly. It's so important to have a strong third eye chakra so that you can see the truth and make good decisions. Your intuition is your strongest ally in this regard.

There are several things you can do to balance your third eye chakra. One is to meditate on the color indigo. Visualize a peaceful indigo light coming from your third eye and filling your entire body with its calming energy. You can even visualize the eye opening up and expanding your field of vision.

Another way to balance your third eye chakra is to spend time in nature. Connecting with the natural world will help you to feel more grounded and centered. Spend time outside, barefoot if possible.

Take deep breaths and let the fresh air fill your lungs. Listen to the birds singing and the leaves rustling in the breeze. Drink in the beauty of nature and let it fill you with peace and calm.

You may also want to try crystal therapy. Crystals like amethyst, sodalite, and lapis lazuli are all great for balancing the third eye chakra. Simply hold the crystal in your hand and focus on its energy.

Crown Chakra

The seventh chakra is the crown chakra. This chakra is located at the top of the head. The crown chakra is associated with spirituality, enlightenment, and connection to the Divine.

The crown chakra is often said to be the most important chakra because it is through this chakra that we connect with our higher selves, our intuition, and our spiritual guidance. Similar to the third eye chakra, the crown chakra is often associated with psychic abilities and extrasensory perception.

When the crown chakra is balanced, we feel connected to our higher purpose and are able to live our lives from a place of intuition and inner knowing. We are also more open to receiving guidance from our spiritual guides. If you find yourself becoming attracted to spiritual practices and metaphysical concepts, it means your crown chakra is opening. A blocked chakra is the result of living in a stressful, fast-paced world where we are disconnected from our true selves.

Signs that your crown chakra is imbalanced include feeling disconnected from your spiritual side, feeling lost or confused about your life purpose, difficulty meditating or connecting with your higher self or a sense of cynicism or skepticism about spirituality. Sometimes people are raised being conditioned to believe that spirituality is not real or that it is only for "woo-woo" people. If this is something you struggle with, it means your crown chakra needs some extra attention.

Healing the crown chakra can be done through meditation, energy work, and connecting with nature, surrounded by the beauty and wonder of the natural world. This helps us to remember our connection to all of life and to the Divine. When meditating, you can imagine a white or violet light entering through the top of your head and filling your entire being with Divine light. This light represents healing, love, and protection.

You can also try affirmations to help balance your crown chakra. Some examples include:

> *"I am connected to my higher self."*
>
> *"I am one with the Divine."*
>
> *"I am guided by my intuition."*
>
> *"I live my life with purpose and meaning."*

Take some time to explore what works best for you and trust that you are being guided to exactly what you need. The most important thing is to have an open mind and heart and to be willing to step out of your comfort zone. Trust that the universe has your back and that you are being supported on your journey.

HOW CHAKRAS AFFECT YOUR INTUITION

Now that we have covered the basics of the chakra system, it's important to understand the relation between the chakras and our intuition. Our chakras can be seen as doors that open us to different aspects of life. When they are blocked or imbalanced, we may have trouble accessing our intuition or connecting with our higher selves.

You can think of your energetic body as a car. If you want to go somewhere, you need to have all the parts in good working order. If your engine is not working, the car won't go. If your battery is dead, the car won't start. In the same way, if our chakras are blocked or imbalanced, we will have trouble accessing our intuition or connecting with our higher selves. If you want to have strong psychic abilities, you need to make sure that all of your chakras are open and balanced.

As you already know, everything is energy. Just because we don't necessarily see the chakras doesn't mean they aren't there. We also don't see the electricity that powers our homes, but we know it's there. This was a challenging concept for me to grasp at first, but once I did, it completely changed my understanding of energy and how it works.

The chakras are energy centers that exist within the subtle body, which is the non-physical aspect of ourselves. The subtle body consists of the mind, emotions, and energy. It is through the subtle body that we experience life on a more spiritual level. If I were to draw a diagram of an empath's energy field, it would look like a big sponge. We absorb the energy of others, whether we want to or not.

This is why it's so important for empaths to protect their energy and boundaries. If we don't, we can easily become overwhelmed and bogged down by external negativity. When our chakras are open and balanced, we are able to receive and process energy in a healthy way. We are also able to connect with our intuition and higher selves more easily.

CHAKRA BALANCING TECHNIQUES

There are many different ways to heal the chakras. I'm going to share some of the most common and effective methods that I have used and know to be helpful.

Energy Work

One of the best ways to heal the chakras is through energy work. This can be done in a variety of ways, such as reiki, healing touch, and other energy healing modalities. Energy work helps to unblock and balance the chakras by clearing away any stagnant or negative energy. You can find a practitioner in your area by doing a quick search online and asking around for recommendations.

The way energy healing works is that it helps to stimulate the flow of energy in the body. This can help to unblock any stagnant energy and encourage balance. When I've had reiki sessions, I always feel lighter and more balanced afterward. The best way I can explain it is that it's like getting a tune-up for your energetic body. It's very gentle and relaxing, and it can be a great way to reduce stress and promote healing.

Crystal Therapy

Crystal therapy is another wonderful way to heal the chakras. Each chakra has a corresponding crystal that can help to unblock and balance it. For example, amethyst is associated with the crown chakra and can help to encourage spiritual connection and intuition. Citrine is associated with the solar plexus chakra and can help to boost self-confidence and promote creativity.

If you have an interest in learning more about crystals and how to use them, I recommend visiting a local metaphysical store or searching online. You can find crystal kits that contain all of the crystals you need for chakra healing.

Crystals can then be placed on the body (either directly on the skin or slightly above it) in the corresponding chakra area. They can also be held in the hand during meditation or placed under the pillow at night. The key is to work with the crystals that you are drawn to and trust your intuition. This is the reason I personally prefer to buy crystals in person, so that I can hold them and see which ones call to me.

Chakra Color Meditation

I find meditation to be one of the most effective ways to heal and balance the chakras. It helps to quiet the mind and allows you to focus on your breath and the present moment. We have full control over our breath, so it's a great way to focus and center yourself when you're feeling off balance. Meditation also helps to connect you with your higher self and intuition. When you meditate on a regular basis, you will start to notice subtle changes in your energy and the way you think and feel.

A simple yet effective way to meditate is to focus on breath and visualization. You can envision where each chakra is located in the body, and imagine its color radiating out from its center point. Starting from the bottom of your spine at the root chakra, slowly move up through each energy center, picturing its color emanating from your body. As you bring these different color placements to your mind, breathe into each one, allowing that particular energy to expand with each breath. Visualize each chakra spinning and glowing brightly.

Affirmations to Balance Your Chakras

Affirmations are positive statements that you can say to yourself on a daily basis to help shift your mindset. If you're looking to improve your selfesteem, for example, you would repeat affirmations such as "I am worthy" or "I am enough." These affirmations help to retrain your brain and change the way you think about yourself.

If you incorporate affirmations into your daily routine, I guarantee you will feel and see a difference in the way you feel and think.

Similarly, you can use affirmations to help balance your chakras. For each chakra, there are affirmations that can help to unblock and heal it. Here are some examples:

Root chakra: *I am safe. I am grounded. I am supported.*

Sacral chakra: *I am creative. I am passionate. I am alive.*

Solar plexus chakra: *I am confident. I am in control of my life. I am worthy.*

Heart chakra: *I am loved. I am compassionate. I am kind.*

Throat chakra: *I am authentic. I am honest. I communicate with ease.*

Third eye chakra: *I trust my intuition. I see the beauty in life. I am connected to the Universe.*

Crown chakra: *I am divine. I am one with all that is. I am at peace.*

After you have finished meditating, sit for a few minutes and notice how you feel. Take a few deep breaths and allow yourself to adjust to the new energy you've brought into your body. Chakra meditation is a great way to bring balance and harmony into your life. It's also very relaxing and can be done anytime, anywhere.

Chakra Healing Chants

Chakra chants are a powerful way to restore balance in your body and mind. By chanting the appropriate mantra for each chakra, you can open, cleanse, and energize your energy centers.

You might've heard of the power of mantras before. A mantra is a sacred word or phrase that has the ability to create change. When you chant a chakra healing mantra, you're vibrating your vocal cords and sending out positive energy into the universe.

The seven chakras are each associated with a different sound frequency. When you chant the correct mantra for each chakra, you're helping to balance your energy and promote healing.

The first time I came across chants was at a yoga class. I'll be honest, at first, it felt a bit strange to be chanting "Om" in a room full of people. But as I continued to chant, I started to feel more relaxed and centered.

There's something really special about the vibration of sound that can help to promote healing. If you're looking for a way to de-stress and balance your chakras, I encourage you to give chanting a try.

Here are the seven chakras and the corresponding mantra for each one.

1. *Root Chakra – LAM Chant*
2. *Sacral Chakra – VAM Chant*
3. *Solar Plexus Chakra – RAM Chant*
4. *Heart Chakra – YAM Chant*
5. *Throat Chakra – HAM Chant*
6. *Third Eye Chakra – OM Chant*
7. *Crown Chakra – AH Chant*

Remember, there is no wrong way to chant. You don't need to be musically inclined (trust me, I'm not) or have a "good" singing voice (nope, not me either). The most important thing is that you're putting your intention into your practice and allowing the sound vibrations to work their magic.

To hear what these chants sound like, I recommend checking out some guided meditations on YouTube. You can then follow along with the video or chant on your own time. We're lucky to live in an era where we have access to so many helpful resources. I hope you enjoy exploring the world of chakra chants. Experiment and see what works best for you!

Yoga Practice

There are many different types of yoga, but they all have the same goal: To unify the body, mind, and spirit. Yoga can be practiced in many different ways, but most often, it involves physical postures (asanas), breath work (pranayama), and meditation. Yoga is a great way to de-stress, ease anxiety, and promote relaxation. It can also help to improve flexibility, build strength, and increase energy levels. It's also beneficial for chakra health!

In yoga, each pose is said to have specific benefits. For example, the Cobra Pose stimulates the root chakra. The Camel Pose opens the heart chakra. And the Lion Pose releases tension from the third eye chakra. There are many different yoga poses, and each one can be beneficial for chakra health. This is where your breath work comes in.

When you focus on your breath while you're in a yoga pose, you're helping to move energy through your body. This is said to help balance the chakras and promote healing. So if you're looking for a way to cleanse and energize your chakras, yoga is definitely worth exploring!

There are plenty of yoga classes available, both inperson and online. If you're new to yoga, I recommend checking out some beginner-friendly classes. Once you get a feel for the basics, you can start practicing at home with the help of books or online resources. There are plenty of free yoga videos available on the Internet. If you have a chance to attend a live class, that's even better! This will give you the opportunity to immerse yourself in the practice and really get the most out of it. The instructor can also give you guidance and support, which is especially helpful if you're new to yoga practice.

CONNECTING WITH YOUR INNER WISDOM

Learning to Trust Your Intuition

Your intuition is your personal GPS system. It's like having a direct hotline to the Divine. It is that inner knowing that we all have access to. It's that little voice inside your head that gives you guidance and nudges you in the right direction. Learning to trust your intuition can be a challenge, especially if you're used to relying on logic and reasoning. But the more you tune in to your intuition, the easier it will be to trust it.

It's important to pay attention to your gut feeling. When you have a gut feeling about something, it's usually your intuition trying to send you a message. If you get a strong feeling about something, even if you can't explain why it's worth listening to. I wish I had a dollar for every time I second-guessed my intuition. I would be a millionaire by now! There've been many situations where I've had a strong feeling about something, but I didn't listen to it. Perhaps because it didn't feel logical, or it wasn't what I wanted to hear. But every time I've ignored my intuition, it's come back to bite me.

When you ignore your GPS and try to take a shortcut, you usually end up getting lost. The same is true for your intuition. If you try to second-guess it or ignore it, you'll only end up making things more difficult for yourself. But when you trust your intuition and follow its guidance, everything seems to fall into place.

I do want to point out that there's a difference between intuition and wishful thinking. Just because you want something to be true doesn't mean it is. So if you're not sure whether something is your intuition or just wishful thinking, ask yourself if it feels light or heavy. Intuition always feels light, even if it's giving you information you don't want to hear. Wishful thinking, on the other hand, feels heavy and stressful. It's usually based on fear and insecurity.

This is where discernment comes in.

Discernment is the ability to distinguish between truth and lies, between what's real and what's not. It's a bit like having x-ray vision. When you have discernment, you can see through people's BS. You can see through their facade and get to the heart of who they really are. This is an invaluable gift, especially when it comes to dealing with difficult people.

Having strong discernment doesn't mean that you're judgmental or critical. It simply means that you're able to see things as they really are. And when you have this ability, it becomes easier to trust your intuition because you know that it's not just your own opinion or bias that's guiding you. The only time I ever second-guess my intuition is when I can't tell if it's coming from a place of love or fear. If it feels light and positive, then I know it's my intuition. But if it feels heavy and negative, then I know it's just my own fear trying to talk me out of something.

The best way to develop your discernment is through meditation. Meditation helps you to quiet your mind and tune in to your inner guidance. It also allows you to get in touch with your authentic self. When you meditate regularly, you become more attuned to your intuitive guidance, and it becomes easier to trust it.

Learning to trust your intuition takes practice. But the more you tune in to it and follow its guidance, the easier it will be. Eventually, it will become second nature. It becomes a compass that you can always rely on, no matter what situation you find yourself in.

THE MAGIC OF AUTOMATIC WRITING

Automatic writing is a great way to channel your intuition and inner wisdom. It's a form of free writing where you let your hand move freely across the page without thinking too much about what you're writing. As you write, you may be surprised at the wisdom that comes through.

Before we dive into automatic writing, it's important to understand that this is a channeling exercise, not a writing exercise. There are no spelling or grammar rules or correct ways to do this.

To channel your intuition, you need to get into a relaxed and receptive state. The best way to do this is after meditation when your mind is quiet and open. You can also do this first thing in the morning before your mind is too cluttered with thoughts.

Once you're in a relaxed state, start writing. I like to set an intention before I begin. For example, you could ask to receive guidance on a specific issue or question that you have. This helps to focus your attention and allows you to receive specific information. For example, you could ask for guidance on a situation relating to your career, your relationships, or your health. Or maybe you'll want some insight on how to make a difficult decision.

But you don't have to do this if you don't want to. You can simply start writing and see what comes through. There are no wrong answers in automatic writing. Just let the words flow through you without judging or censoring them. The goal is to get out of your own way and allow your intuition to speak through you.

If you find your mind starting to wander, just refocus your attention on your question or on the page in front of you. And if you get stuck, keep writing until something comes through. In the beginning, it might feel somewhat awkward or even forced. But the more you practice automatic writing, the easier it will become. Write whatever comes into your mind, even if it doesn't make sense. Keep your hand moving across the page, and don't worry about what you're writing.

It may help to set a timer for 10-15 minutes so that you don't have to worry about the time. Let yourself write until the timer goes off. Once you're finished, take a few minutes to read over what you've written. Chances are some of it will first sound like gibberish. But as you read through it, you will start to see some valuable insights emerge. You may be surprised at the wisdom that comes through.

LEARNING TO READ AURAS

You might've heard the expression, "He gives off good vibes" or "She has a bad aura about her." These expressions are referring to the energy field that surrounds them.

Auras can also be described as a "mental body" or an "astral body." An aura is made up of electromagnetic energy of different frequencies. In spirituality books, auras are often illustrated as colorful light around the head and body. Aura colors can reveal information about your thoughts, feelings, and health.

The seven layers of the aura are often described as being like the layers of an onion. The physical body is in the middle, surrounded by increasingly ethereal layers. Auras are not typically visible to the naked eye. However, some people are able to see auras by training their eyes to see beyond the physical world. Aura colors can reveal information about your thoughts, feelings, and health. When we are upbeat and happy, our auras tend to be brighter and lighter in color. When we are feeling low, our auras can appear smudged or darker.

For example, a blue aura might represent peace, serenity, and calm. A yellow aura might represent happiness, intellect, and creativity. An orange aura might represent enthusiasm, adventure, and courage. A red aura might represent passion, energy, and strength. A dark or smirk aura might represent fear, anger, or sadness.

I encourage you to experiment with seeing auras for yourself. It's a fun and fascinating way to develop your psychic abilities!

Aura Reading Exercises

If you're interested in learning how to read auras, there are a few things you can do to start training your eyes to see them. One method is to ask someone to stand in front of a white wall. Then focus your gaze on their head and shoulders. Practice using a "soft gaze." This means you're not staring, but rather, you're letting your eyes relax and take in the person's energy field. Initially, you might be able to spot a subtle white light around the person's head. With practice, people report starting to see other colors in their aura. Another exercise is to hold your hand up in front of you and look at it closely. Again, use a soft gaze and relax your eyes. You may start to see a faint outline of color around your hand.

You can also practice observing people around you and see if you can pick up on any colors. With time and practice, you'll become better at it. Just be careful not to stare at people for too long!.

An aura reading can give you insights into your own thoughts, feelings, and behaviors. It can also reveal things about other people. As you become more familiar with aura reading, you'll develop your own intuitive understanding of the colors and their meanings.

I've noticed that people with high levels of energy tend to have brighter auras. For example, I once saw the aura of a woman who was eight months pregnant. She literally had a glow around her! Her aura was a beautiful, bright white light. I could feel her pregnancy energy as a strong, yet gentle, presence. On the other hand, I've also seen people with darker auras who seem to be carrying a lot of negative energy. These individuals can be more challenging to be around and may even drain your own energy levels if you're not careful.

If you're having trouble seeing auras, don't fret! Most are either born with the gift or develop it over time and practice through meditation and energy work. Personally, I sense auras more than I see them. I feel the energy of a person's aura as a subtle sensation in my body. However, every now and then, I'll catch a glimpse of an aura's colors out of the corner of my eye.

Just remember that it takes time and practice to develop your intuition. So don't get discouraged if you don't see results right away. With a little patience and perseverance, you'll be able to pick up on the energy of the world around you. And developing your intuitive abilities is a never-ending journey that can be incredibly eye-opening and rewarding!

CONNECTING WITH YOUR SPIRIT GUIDES

Your spirit guides are non-physical beings of light who are here to offer you guidance, support, and love. They are your personal cheerleaders and have your best interests at heart. Like your spiritual allies who want nothing more than for you to succeed. So how do you connect with them? The most important thing is to be open to receiving their guidance. It can be as simple as asking your guides for help with specific problems or challenges you're facing and trusting that they will lead you in the right direction.

There were two scenarios in my life that led me to start working on my spirit guides. The first was when I had very little knowledge of them. As a newly engaged couple, my husband and I were traveling through Spain. It was a beautiful fall afternoon as we were taking pictures and strolling through a park. The ground was completely covered in a carpet of multicolored leaves that were crunching under our feet. The whole scene felt magical, like in a romantic love story. "I have a brilliant idea for a photo!" I told my husband. I then picked up a big handful of leaves from the ground and threw them up in the air, as an ecstatic three-year-old would. I envisioned a stunning photo of them fluttering down around us like colorful confetti.

And down like confetti they went. And so did the engagement ring off my finger. The result was an awkward-looking selfie of me with a pile of leaves stuck to my head and a look of horror on my face... I was devastated and so embarrassed that I had lost such an important piece of jewelry. I thought my husband would want to file for a divorce before he even had a chance to marry me.

It also didn't help that the ring was designed in two pieces that fit together. Even if we found one part, the ring would be useless without the other. I immediately started tearing through the leaves, frantically searching for the ring. My poor fiancé tried his best to dig through the leaves to search for it. But after 20 minutes of meticulous digging and crawling around on all fours, it became clear that it was hopeless. The ring was gone. I felt like such a klutz!

Then, I remembered reading about spirit guides in a random book I'd picked up at a library. I composed myself and decided to ask my spirit guides for help. And sure enough, within minutes, my husband found the first half. Can you believe it? A few minutes later, a kind Brazilian couple approached us in sympathy and offered to help. To make a long story short, they had found the other half of the ring that had somehow bounced on the fence and landed across the street! I couldn't believe our luck. We were so grateful to have found it and even more grateful for the help of our kind strangers and spirit guides. That was the first time I experienced the true magic of connecting with my guides. The rest is history!

The second time was when I was about to give birth to our second child. I had a scheduled C-section, my contractions were getting stronger, and I was getting more and more nervous about the surgery. To make matters worse, the epidural wasn't working as it should, and I was starting to feel nauseous. The doctors informed me that if the next shot of epidural didn't kick in, I would have to be put under general anesthesia for the surgery.

That was my absolute worst-case scenario. I didn't want to be put to sleep and miss the birth of my child. The whole situation felt out of control. At that moment, I again asked for guidance from my spirit guides. I visualized them surrounding me, infusing me with strength and support. And sure enough, within seconds, I started to feel more relaxed and centered. Magically, the epidural finally kicked in. Instead of feeling scared, I felt confident and prepared. Giving birth is always an intense experience, but with the help of my guides, it was also one of the most beautiful moments of my life. The surgery went without a hitch, and our beautiful baby girl was born healthy and happy. I recall the doctors being in awe of how calm and relaxed I was throughout the whole ordeal. To be honest, even I was surprised at how well things had gone. But I knew it was due to the help of my spirit guides.

These are just two examples of how your spirit guides can offer you guidance, support, and love when you need it most. So if you're ever feeling lost, confused, or alone, just know that your guides are always there for you, ready to help in whatever way they can. Just be open to receiving their guidance, and you'll be amazed at the ways they can help you transform your life for the better.

I wanted to share these examples to illustrate that you don't need to follow any fancy rituals or be a super spiritual person to connect with your guides. It can be as simple as just asking them for help and being open to receiving it.

ASKING FOR SIGNS

Guides can communicate with us in many ways, but one of the most common is through signs. If you're wondering if your guides are trying to tell you something, pay attention to any repeating numbers you see, such as 11:11, 222, or 333. They often pop up when we're on the right track or need confirmation from our guides that we're headed in the right direction.

You might also start seeing certain animals or symbols more frequently. For example, if you've been considering a major life change and you keep seeing images of a butterfly, it could be a sign from your guides that it's time for you to spread your wings and make a transformation.

Pay attention to the synchronicities and everyday miracles that occur around you. These are often messages from your guides. You might start to see the same number repeatedly, or you might hear a song on the radio that seems to be speaking directly to you. Trust your intuition and follow the guidance you receive.

For example, I keep seeing the number 1111. I see it multiple times a day. On my phone. On license plates. On the clock... it appears everywhere. So I asked my guides what it meant. And I received the guidance that it's a signal for me to keep moving forward on my dreams and goals because I'm on the right path. If you're not sure how to interpret a sign you've received, just ask your guides for clarification. They're always happy to help.

Another way to connect with your spirit guides is through visualization exercises. One of my favorites is to imagine yourself walking through a door into their realm. It's a beautiful place full of love and light, and your guides are there waiting to greet you with open arms. As you spend time in this realm, allow their energy to infuse you with strength, courage, and wisdom. Then, when you're ready, imagine yourself walking back through the door into the physical world. Bring whatever guidance or insights you received back with you and allow them to guide you in your everyday life.

You can also connect with your guides during your meditation practice. One way to do this is through the automatic writing exercise I shared earlier. Before you start writing, ask your guides to come in and give you guidance on the issue or question you're working on. Then start writing and see what comes through. When you quiet your mind, it becomes easier to hear their whispers of guidance. You can ask your guides to help you with protecting your energy and developing your psychic abilities as well. They can help you release any old patterns or beliefs that are no longer serving you, shield you from negative energy, and give you the strength to stand in your power.

There are endless ways to work with your guides. Trust that they are always there for you, ready to help in whatever way they can. And know that you are never alone.

CONCLUSION

As you embrace your empathy and psychic abilities, you will begin to notice positive changes in your life. More and more, you will trust your intuition and make decisions based on your own inner knowledge. You will find yourself better able to handle relationships, both personal and professional. Your communication with others will improve, and you will understand their needs and feelings. You'll also feel empowered to help others through your compassion, guidance, and wisdom. With practice, you will become more skilled in using them and discover just how far they can take you. Trust your intuition, follow your heart, and let your empathy and psychic powers guide you to a happier, more fulfilling life.

CONCLUSION

In a world that can be harsh and overwhelming at times, your empathy and psychic abilities are your superpowers. They give you the ability to feel and see things that others can't. To know things that others don't. And with this knowledge comes power. The power to make a difference. The power to change the world.

When our society is faced with problems, it is often the empaths who are the first to step up and offer help. Who see beyond the surface and into the heart of the matter. And who are brave enough to use their abilities to make a positive difference.

Empathy and psychic abilities are about understanding people and emotions, being compassionate and kind, and using your intuition to guide you through life. So embrace your abilities. Develop them. Nurture them. And let them guide you on your journey through life. They were given to you for a reason. To be a light in the darkness and a force of good in the world. Simply by being true to your authentic self, you can inspire, guide, and support others to do the same.

Never doubt your abilities or let anyone tell you that you are too sensitive. Your sensitivity is a quality to be celebrated! You are exactly who you are supposed

CONCLUSION

to be. An intuitive empath. A gifted individual with the power to make a difference. Your sensitivity, insights, and compassion make you uniquely qualified to create positive change in the world.

I hope this book sparked a light inside of you. That it reminded you of your own innate gifts and inspired you to seek further knowledge and develop your talents. There is so much potential for positive change when you embrace your empathy and intuition. Thank you for being a part of that journey with me. Together, we can spread healing, love, and light throughout the planet.

The world needs your light. It's time to shine!

LET'S CONNECT!

Join our Facebook group to connect with empaths from all over the world who are dedicated to learning, developing, and empowering one another.

BIBLIOGRAPHY

Bam, N. N. (2021, December 9). *Understanding 7 Types of Empaths*. Goodnet. Retrieved January 6, 2022, from https://www.goodnet.org/articles/understanding-7-types-empaths

Blair, M. (2021, October 6). *11 Essential Rules Every Empath Needs to Know*. Yoga Journal. Retrieved June 12, 2022, from https://www.yogajournal.com/lifestyle/12-essential-rules-everyempath-needs-to-know/

Brady, K. (2020, November 11). *Being An Empath: The Benefits*. Keir Brady Counseling Services. Retrieved June 6, 2022, from https://keirbradycounseling.com/empath-benefits/

Davis, F. (2021, February 2). *10 Crystals for Intuition & Psychic Ability: Tap Into Your Innate Power*. Cosmic Cuts. Retrieved June 23, 2022, from https://cosmiccuts.com/en-ca/blogs/healing-stones-blog/crystals-for-intuition-psychic-ability

Firestone, L. (2017, September 16). *Empaths: Is being an empath a superpower or a super-stressor?* PsychAlive. Retrieved June 1, 2022, from https://www.psychalive.org/empaths

Greenberg, R. (2017, November 14). *Avoiding Emotional Overload When You're Highly Empathetic*. Tiny Buddha. Retrieved June 21, 2022, from https://tinybuddha.com/blog/how-to-overcome-emotional-overload-when-youre-highly-empathetic/

Kelly, A. (2018, July 2). *Am I Psychic? How to Tap Into Your Own Psychic Abilities*. Allure. Retrieved June 6, 2022, from https://www.allure.com/story/am-i-psychic-how-to-tap-intopsychic-abilities

Kind Earth. (2020a, August 5). *7 Boundary Exercises for Empaths and Sensitive People*. Retrieved June 19, 2022, from https://

www.kindearth.net/7-boundary-exercises-for-empaths-andother-sensitive-people/

Kind Earth. (2020b, August 15). *The importance of grounding for empaths and sensitive people*. Retrieved June 19, 2022, from https://www.kindearth.net/the-importance-of-groundingfor-empaths-and-sensitive-people/

Kind Earth. (2021, January 25). *Compassionate Eating for Empaths and Highly Sensitive People*. Retrieved June 22, 2022, from https://www.kindearth.net/compassionate-eating-forempaths-and-highly-sensitive-people/

Leppington, M. (2022, May 25). *21 Crystals For Intuition: The Essential Guide*. Conscious Items. Retrieved June 24, 2022, from https://consciousitems.com/blogs/practice/crystalsfor-intuition

Little Yellow Dot. (2019, May 17). *Water and the Empath*. Retrieved June 22, 2022, from https://www.littleyellowdot.com/water-and-the-empath/

LonerWolf. (2022, January 11). *Automatic Writing: How to Channel Your Soul's Wisdom*. Retrieved June 26, 2022, from https://lonerwolf.com/automatic-writing/

Markowitz, D. (2017, October 28). *The Best Diet for Empaths and Highly Sensitive Persons*. Dave Markowitz. Retrieved June 20, 2022, from https://www.davemarkowitz.com/blog/36/The-Best-Diet-for-Empaths-and-Highly-Sensitive-Persons/

mindbodygreen. (2021a, August 16). *Think You Could Be An Empath? 12 Signs To Watch Out For & What It Really Means*. Retrieved June 2, 2022, from https://www.mindbodygreen.com/articles/empath

mindbodygreen. (2021b, October 29). *A Beginner's Guide To The 7 Chakras*. Retrieved June 25, 2022, from https://www.mindbodygreen.com/0-91/The-7-Chakras-for-Beginners.html

mindbodygreen. (2021c, December 17). *How To Use Your Intuition Like A Professional Psychic*. Retrieved June 7, 2022, from https://www.mindbodygreen.com/articles/the-4-types-ofintuition-and-how-to-tap-into-each

Myles, A. (2017, June 28). *The Top 10 Truths & Myths about Empaths*. Elephant Journal. Retrieved June 6, 2022, from https://www.elephantjournal.com/2017/05/the-top-10truths-myths-about-empaths/

Northrup, C. (2018, March 21). *8 Ways to Turn Your Empathy into A Super Power*. Christiane Northrup. Retrieved June 10, 2022, from https://www.drnorthrup.com/8-ways-to-turn-yourempathy-into-a-super-power/

Orloff, B. J., MD. (2017, July 20). *Judith Orloff MD 4 Signs You Might Be an Intuitive Empath*. Oprah.Com. Retrieved June 9, 2022, from https://www.oprah.com/inspiration/judithorloff-md-4-signs-you-might-be-an-intuitive-empath

Orloff, J. (2021a, May 21). *5 Protection Strategies for Empaths*. Judith Orloff. Retrieved June 11, 2022, from https://drjudithorloff.com/5-protection-strategies-for-empaths-2/

Orloff, J. (2021b, September 8). *Reasons Why People Become Empaths: From Trauma to Genetics*. Judith Orloff MD. Retrieved June 2, 2022, from https://drjudithorloff.com/4reasons-why-people-become-empaths-from-trauma-togenetics/

Ottewell, C. (2021, December 17). *Spiritual Protection - Using Essential Oils for Spiritual Wellbeing*. The Oily Witch. Retrieved June 22, 2022, from https://www.theoilywitch.co.uk/essential-oils/spiritual-protection

Psychological and Educational Consulting. (2020, March 5). *The Difference Between Highly Sensitive People and Empaths*. Retrieved June 3, 2022, from https://www.psychedconsult.com/the-difference-between-highly-sensitive-people-andempaths/

Quintana, A. (2021, April 11). *Empath Environments: How to Create a Sanctuary that Supports You*. Holistic Fashionista.

Retrieved June 24, 2022, from https://www.holisticfashionista.com/lifestyle-guide/all/empath-environments-how-tocreate-a-sanctuary-that-supports-you

Shour, E. (2021, May 3). *10 Essential Oils For Protection Against Negative Energy*. BoomBoom Naturals. Retrieved June 24, 2022, from https://boomboomnaturals.com/blogs/news/essential-oils-protection-against-negative-energy

Smith, M. R. (n.d.). *How to Prevent Sleep Problems for Empaths*. Empath Connection. Retrieved June 21, 2022, from https://www.empathconnection.com/post/empaths-absorb-energywhile-sleeping

Stelter, G. (2016, December 19). *A Beginner's Guide to the 7 Chakras and Their Meanings*. Healthline. Retrieved June 25, 2022, from https://www.healthline.com/health/fitness-exercise/7-chakras#:%7E:text=Chakra%20(cakra%20in%20Sanskrit)%20means,emotional%20and%20physical%20well%2Dbeing.

Tiggelen, A. (2021, November 30). *The Ultimate Guide To Visualization For Empaths*. HiSensitives. Retrieved June 15, 2022, from https://hisensitives.com/blog/visualization-empathsguide/

Tiny Rituals. (n.d.). *14 Crystals For Empaths: Release Your Power & Ground Yourself*. Retrieved June 22, 2022, from https://tinyrituals.co/blogs/tiny-rituals/14-crystals-for-empathsrelease-your-power-ground-yourself

Valko, L. (2021, January 8). *14 Things Empaths Absolutely Need in Life to Be Happy*. Highly Sensitive Refuge. Retrieved June 20, 2022, from https://highlysensitiverefuge.com/14-thingsempaths-need-in-life-to-be-happy/

Printed in Great Britain
by Amazon